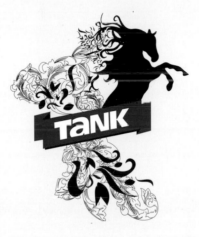

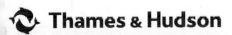
Thames & Hudson

Edited by Masoud Golsorkhi and Andreas Laeufer

Tank
T +44 (0)20 7434 0110
F +44 (0)20 7434 9232
www.tankmagazine.com

First published in 2006 in paperback in the United States of America by
Thames & Hudson Inc., 500 Fifth Avenue, New York, New York 10110

thamesandhudsonusa.com

Library of Congress Catalog Card Number 2005906280

ISBN-13: 978-0-500-28597-8
ISBN-10: 0-500-28597-7

Printed and bound in China by Imago

IANK I00

contents

INTRODUCTION

by Charlotte Cotton

Photographers have perhaps never been as self-conscious as they are today, so aware of the impact, cultural reception and means of dissemination of their imagery. In the exaggerated, oppositional terms of our age, two key modes of photographic practice come into play.

The first is in the realm of galleries and anywhere photography is presented unequivocally as an art form. There, the prevalent tempo is consciously, respectfully slow. Prints of large sizes and high production values declare a system that privileges aesthetics and processes that connote protracted care and scrutiny. The second finds purest expression in the editorial and advertising pages of glossy magazines, where the regulated, market-informed popular visualizations of our era are found. While their subjects often differ, both modes share the significant extent to which the final context of page or wall defines a given photograph's substance and meaning.

No one who wishes photography well could consider these differentiated, prestigious contexts the beginning of the end of the medium. But it would take a naïve soul to think that these contexts constitute the scope of what photography can mean. If we concentrate on only those images deemed most media-worthy in recent years, we surrender to a cultural amnesia about the diversity of photographic creativity through its history. Since when has this sensitive medium, whose makers can be so precise in their ideas and visions yet whose audience is so broad, been allied exclusively to dominant commercial forces? The answer to this question is never.

Photography's position today may be qualified by the twin lenses of art and advertising, but the power of photography will always lie in its capacity both to function within and to contradict the contexts in which it reaches the public realm. The magazine itself was, in the twentieth century, a site where ideas from the profound to the light-hearted, from the long-gestated to the rapidly reflexive, found a home.

Tank is one of the few independent, risk-taking, pluralistic vehicles for what actually constitutes photography today. If you seek a checklist of the known, already validated photographic styles and names, or the fashions, bodies and societal narratives with which you are already comfortable, Tank is not for you. What you will find here is the experimental truth – the belief – that photographers predict rather than reflect what is meaningful in our culture. It is rare and special to have a magazine that holds to a value system that counters the current direction of magazine publishing

Tank functions as an antidote to the nagging feeling that we have entered an age in which advertising and editorial are indistinguishable in both style and message; to the suspicion that writing that analyzes, rather than markets, contemporary culture is a lost art. Tank has commissioned bravely – outside the small roster of photographers and stylists that at any one time determines the mainstream narratives of fashion. Tank achieves what so few magazines aim for or even attempt: to be gorgeously glossy and widely distributed yet still maintain an independent point of view. There is also a sense of the magazine's commitment to publishing photographic projects that it recognizes, ahead of the game, as revealing markers of our age. It is more than simply a willingness to publish independent photographic practice. It is an attitude towards magazine publishing that believes the page is the platform for photographic ideas rather than the message in and of itself. This distinction is easily missed because of the short shelf life of a magazine. But, here, in this second volume collected from its past pages, Tank's unique perspective is plain to see and is to be saluted.

What is a magazine?

What makes a magazine a magazine?

Does it have to be a certain size?

What should it contain?

Should it put art next to fashion next to architecture and diaries and fiction?

Should it be instantly disposable or about preservation for posterity?

Should it be about information or contemplation?

How should it address its readers?

Should it make them feel like excluded outsiders or should it be like their cleverest friend?

Should it be knowing or should it be searching?

Should it be elitist or should it be for everyone?

Should it tell untold stories in untold ways, or should it stick to saying the same thing in different ways?

How can it be exclusive and inclusive at the same time?

What sort of a name is Tank anyway?

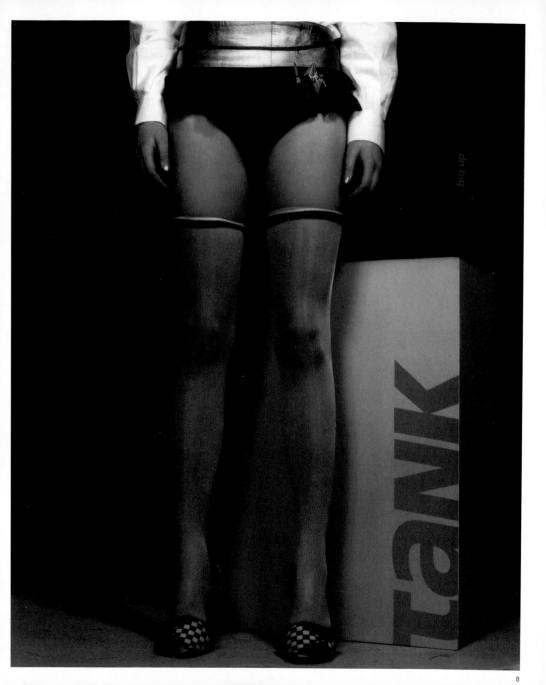

BETTER IS BIGGER

VOLUME 2 · ISSUE 1 · DECEMBER 2000 · COVER PHOTOGRAPH BY GILLES TOLÉDANO

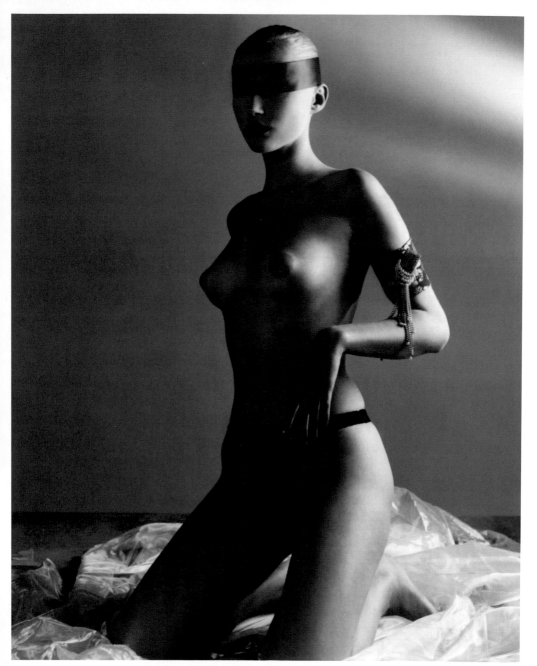

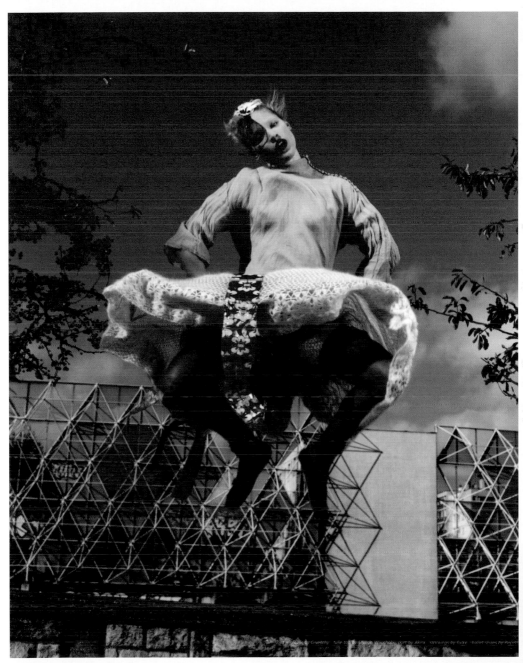

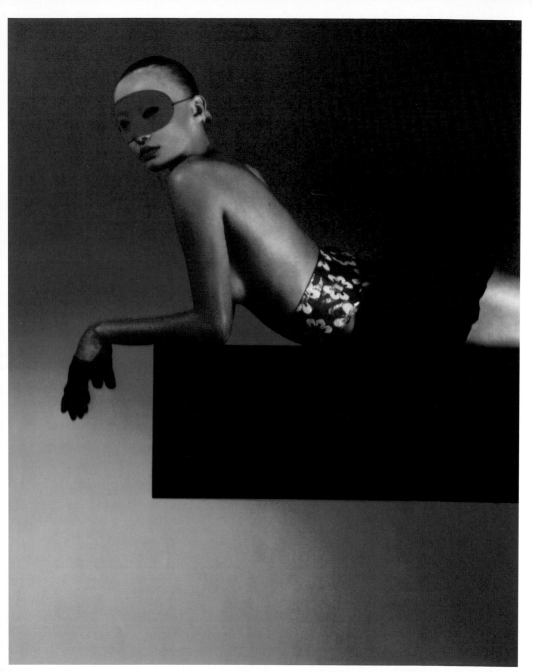

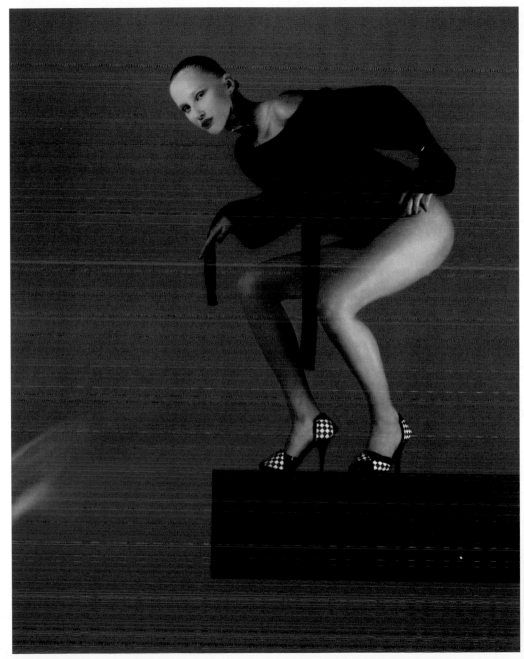

MARGARET SALMON + DEAN WIAND

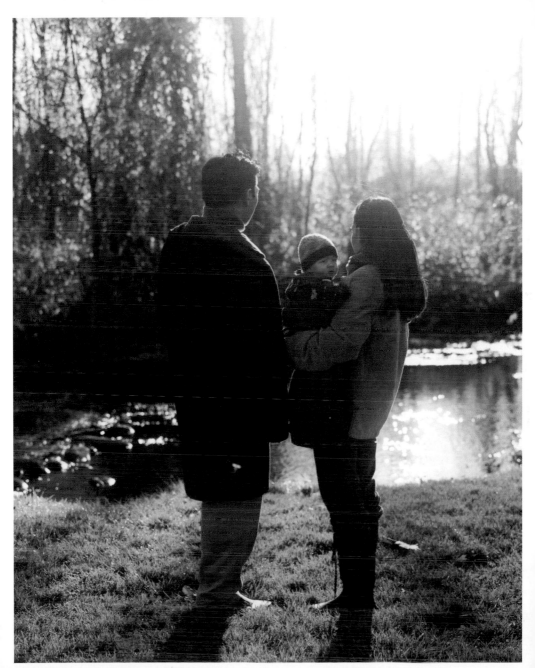

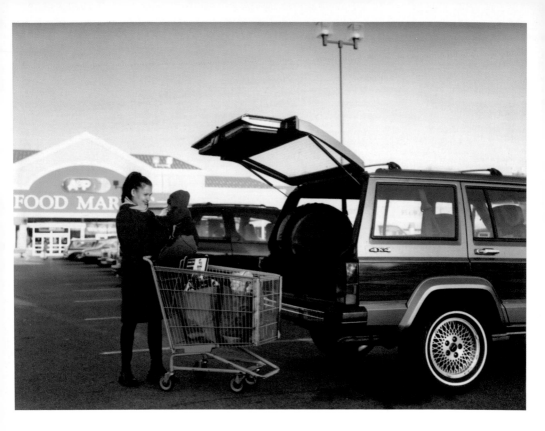

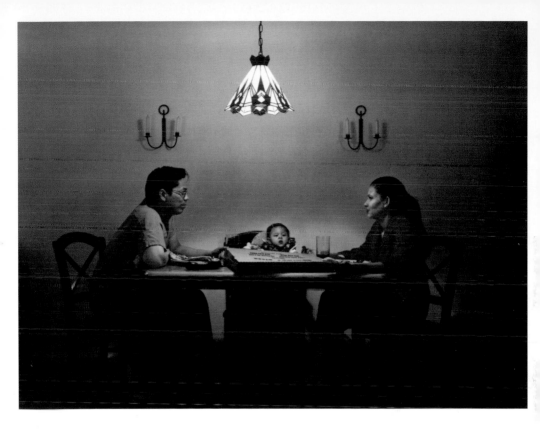

ALI MAHDAVI

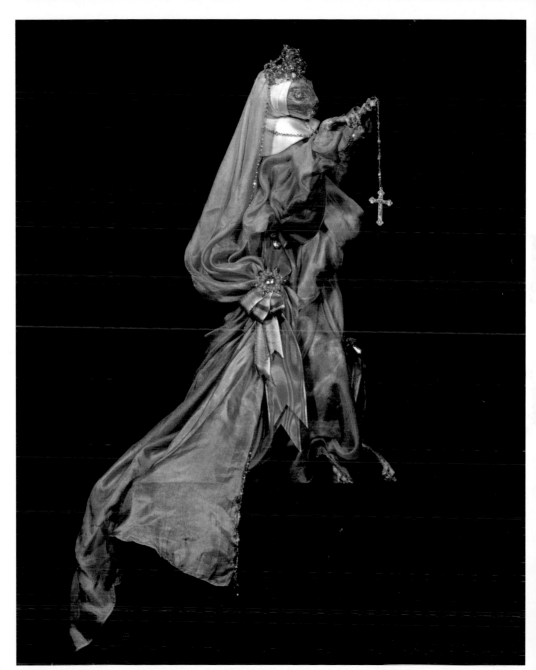

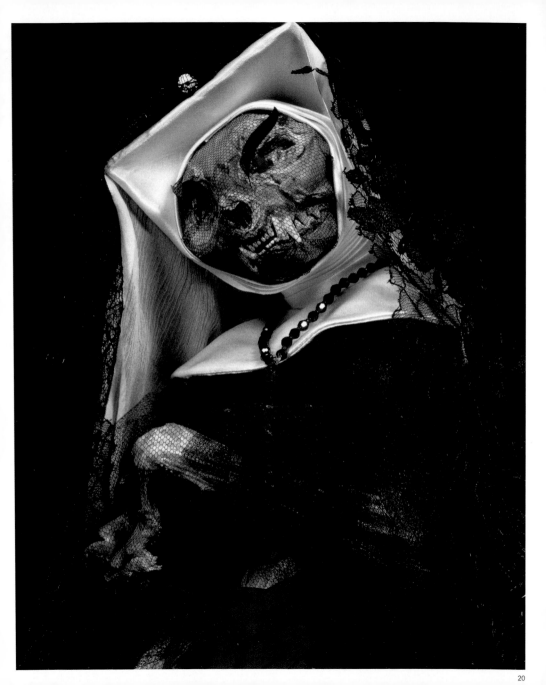

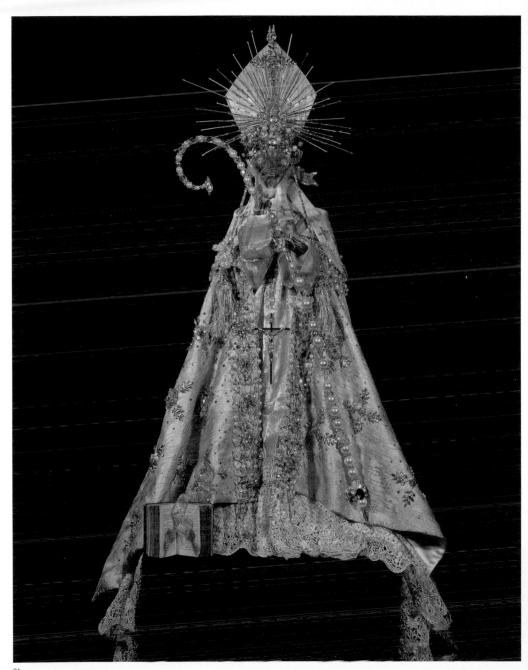

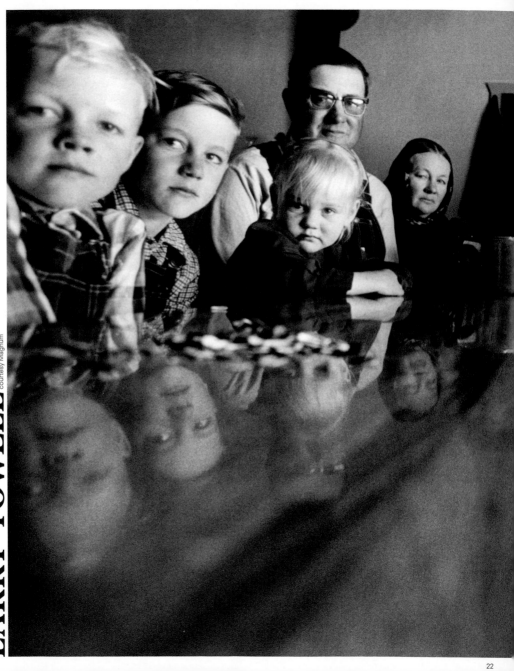

 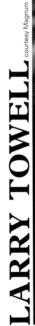 courtesy Magnum

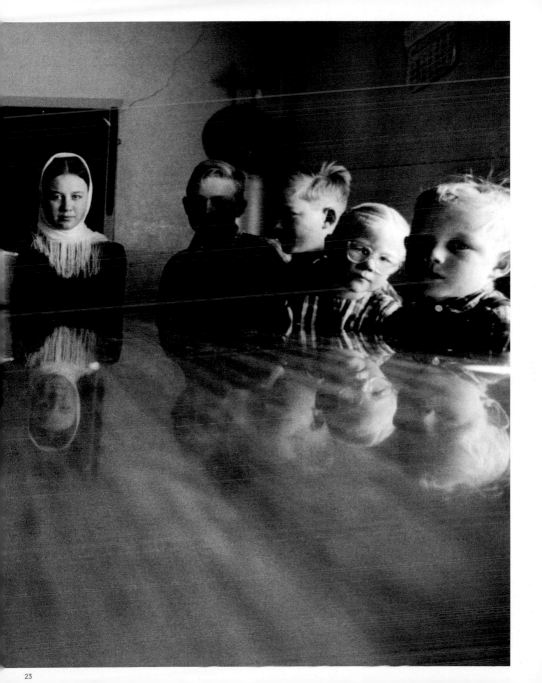

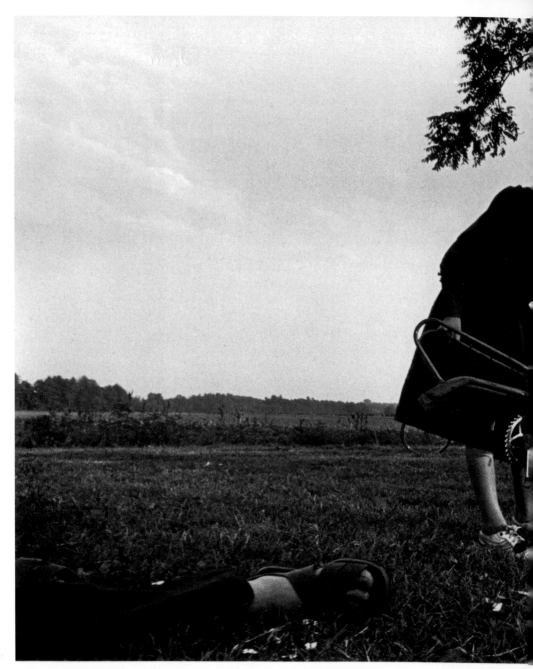

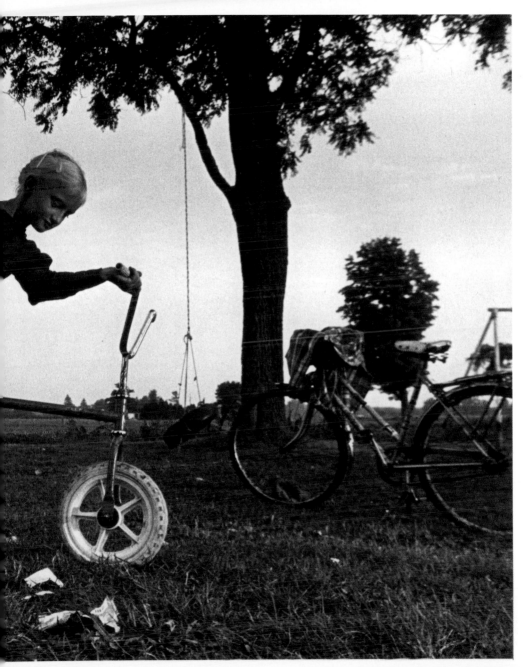

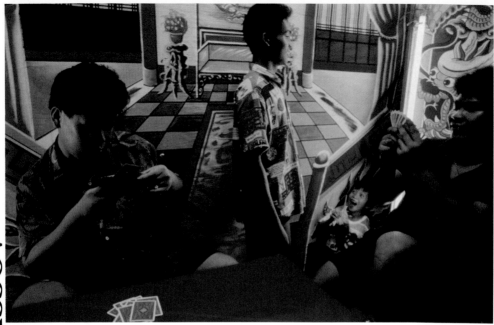

GUEORGUI PINKHASSOV

courtesy Magnum

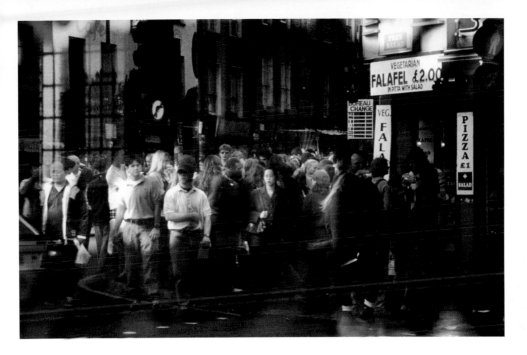

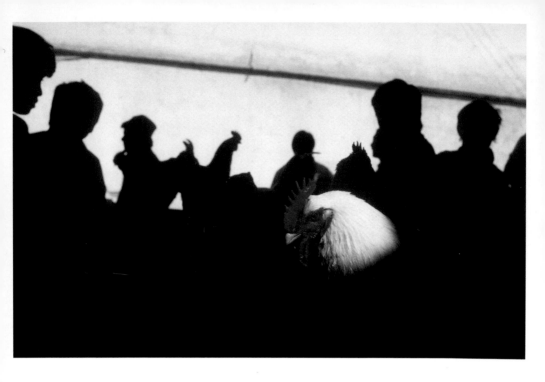

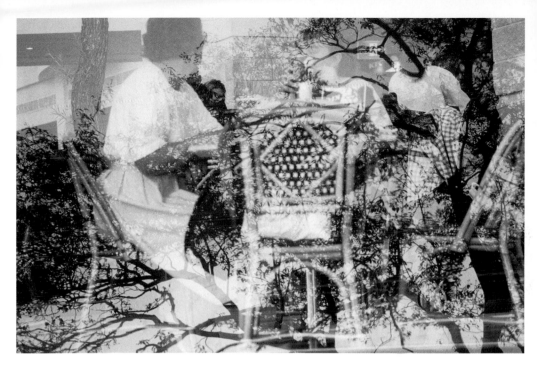

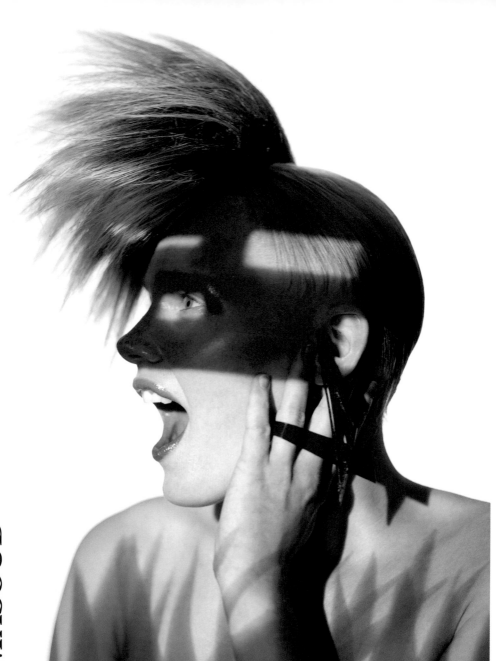

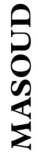
MASOUD

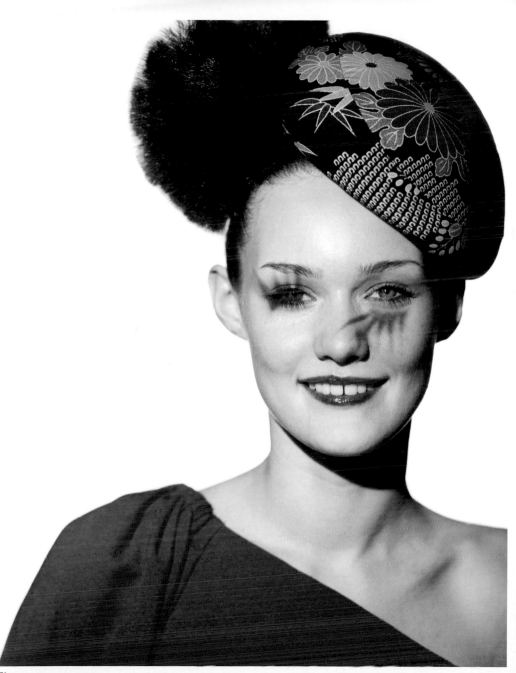

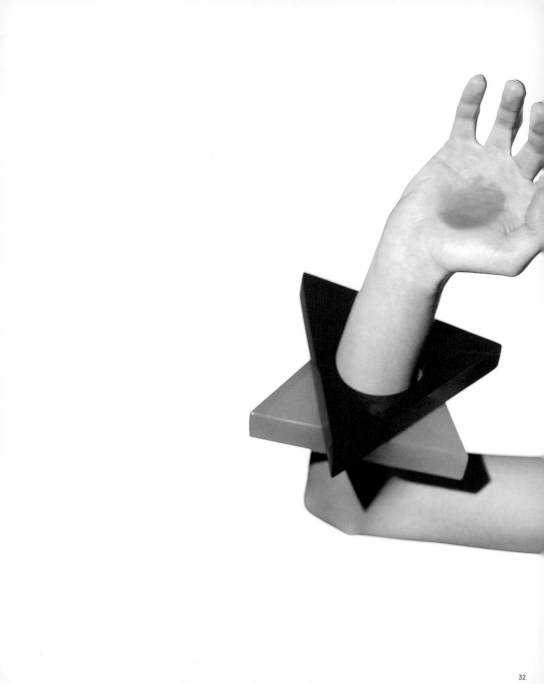

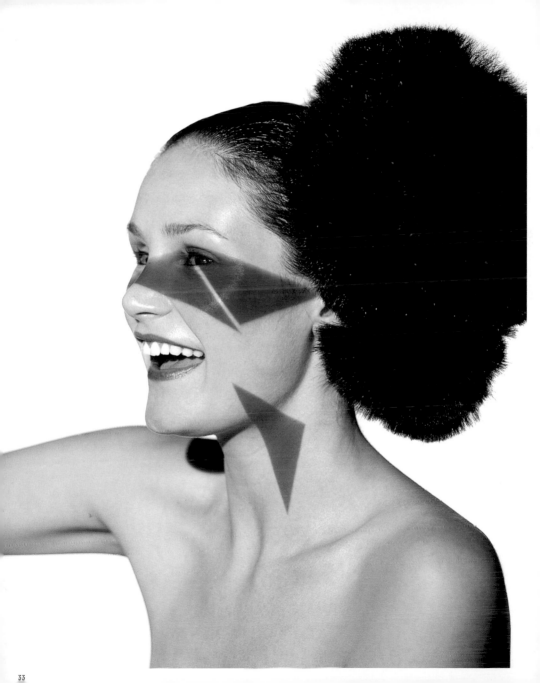

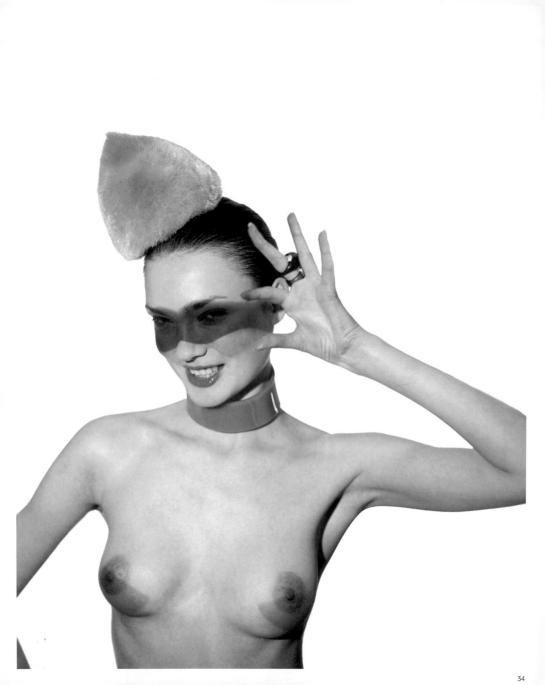

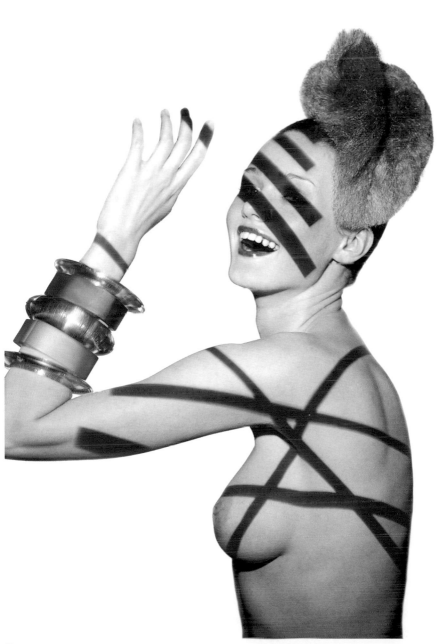

JOHN-PAUL PIETRUS

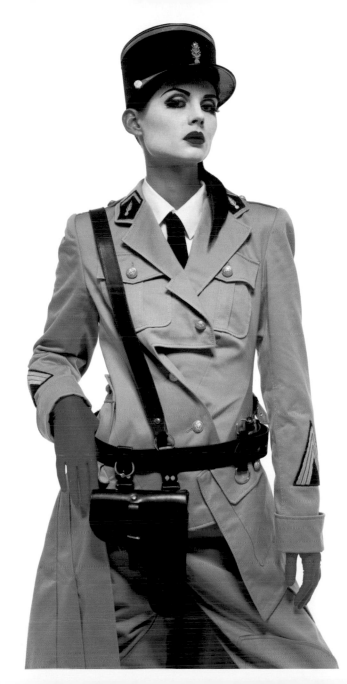

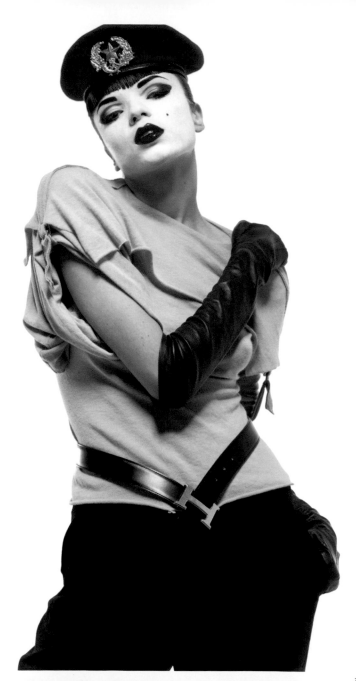

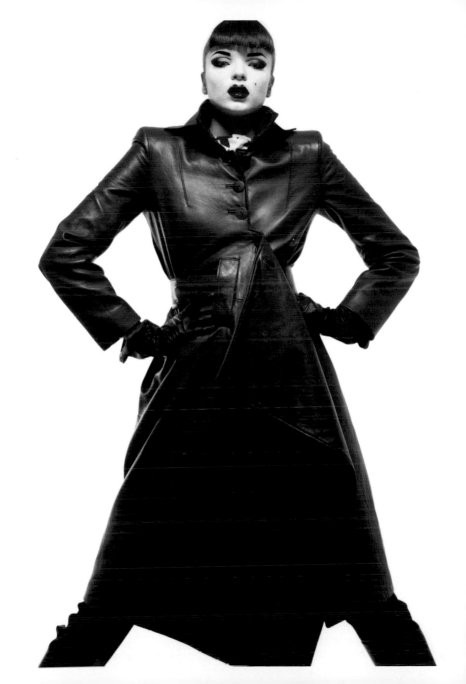

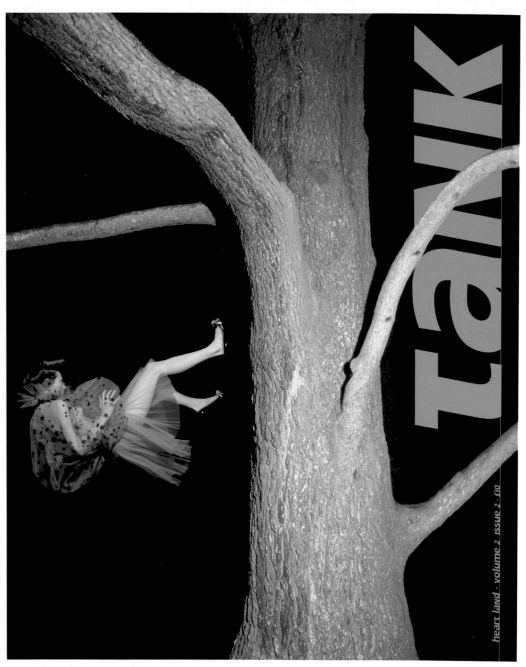

TANK

heart land · volume 2 · issue 2 · £10

EVERGREEN

VOLUME 2 · ISSUE 2 · FEBRUARY 2001 · COVER PHOTOGRAPH BY PATRICK JAMES MICHEL

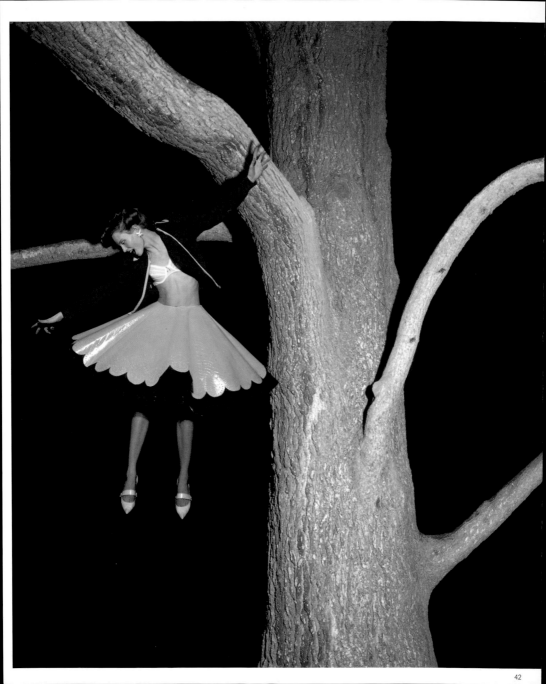

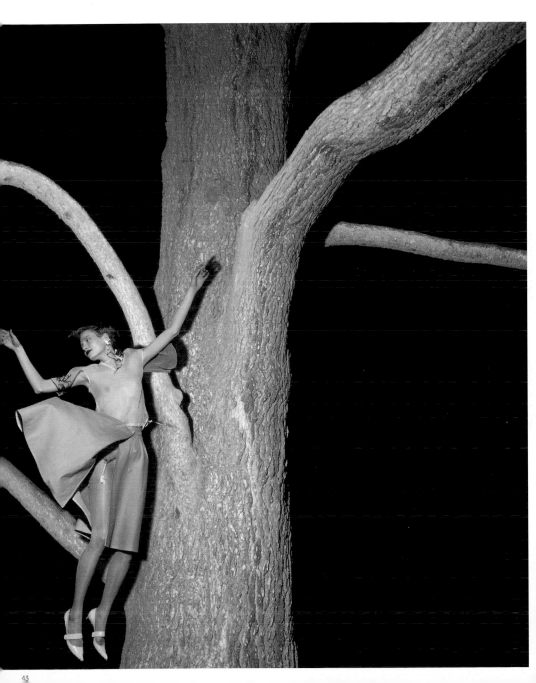

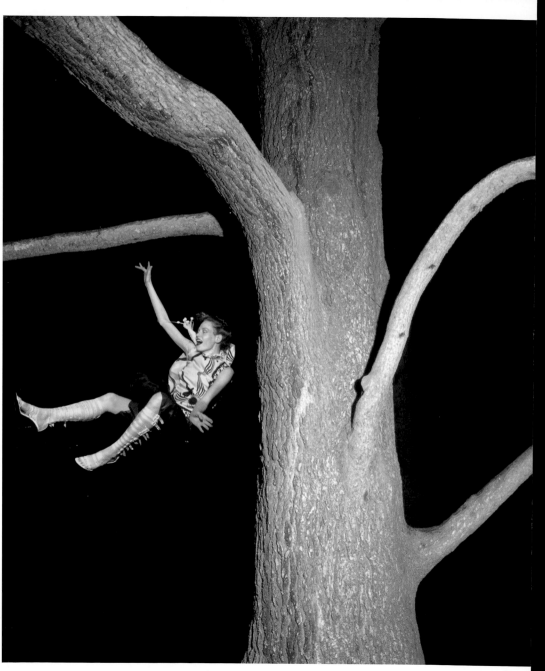

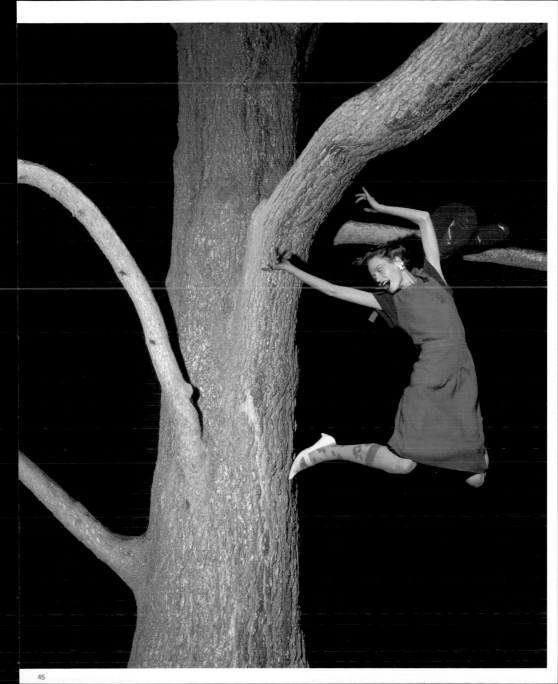

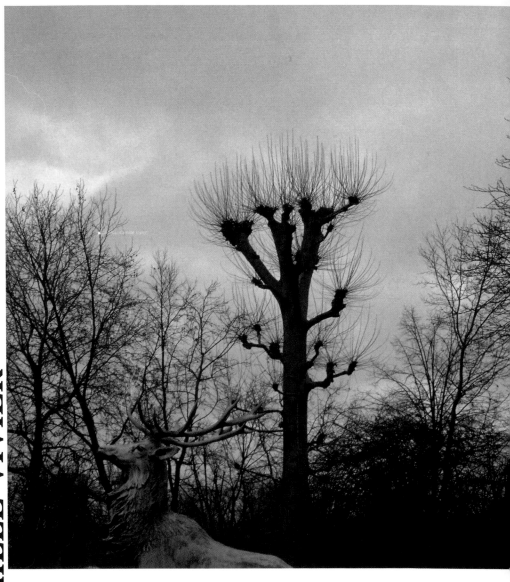

CAMILLE VIVIER

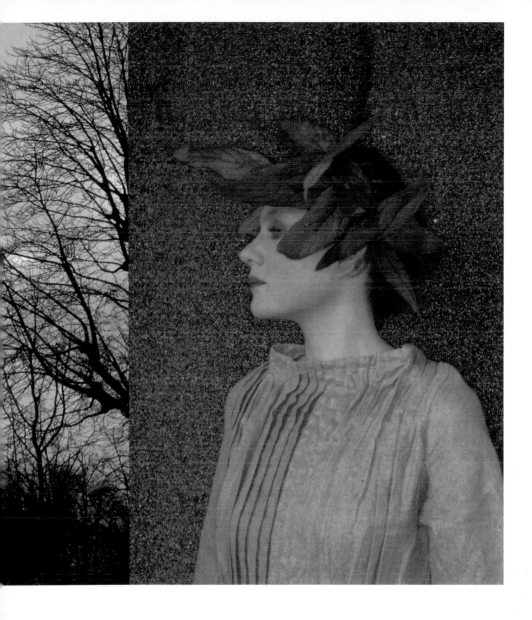

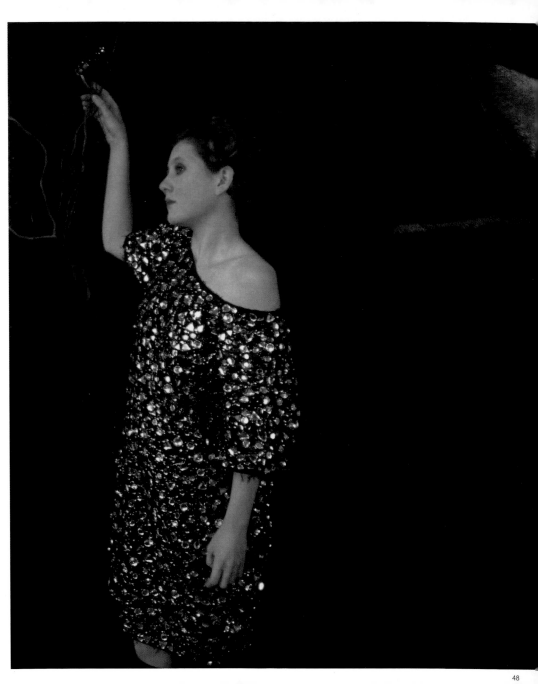

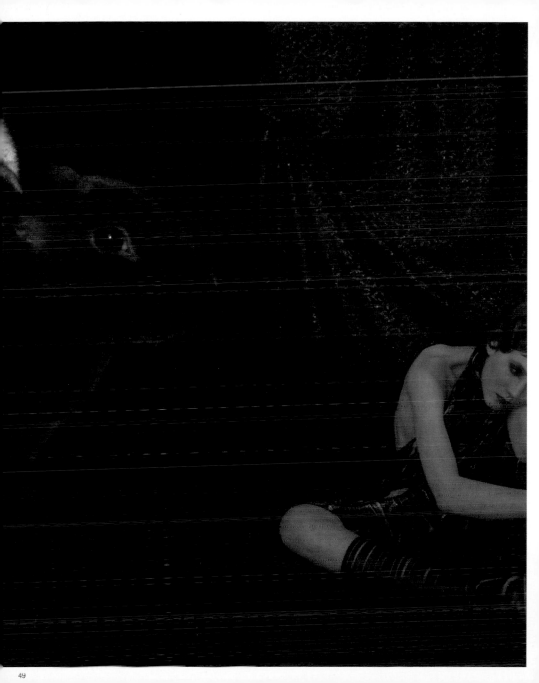

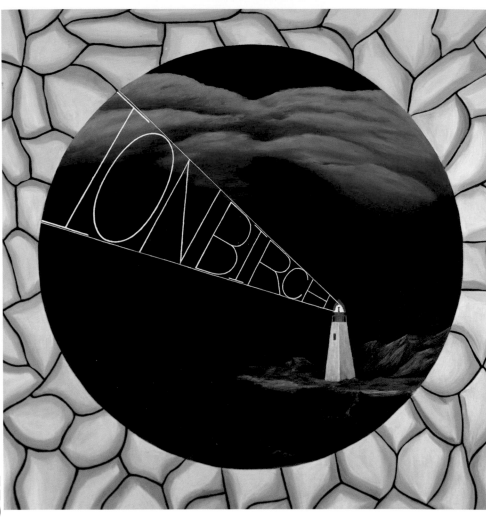

ION BIRCH
courtesy Bronwyn Keenan Gallery

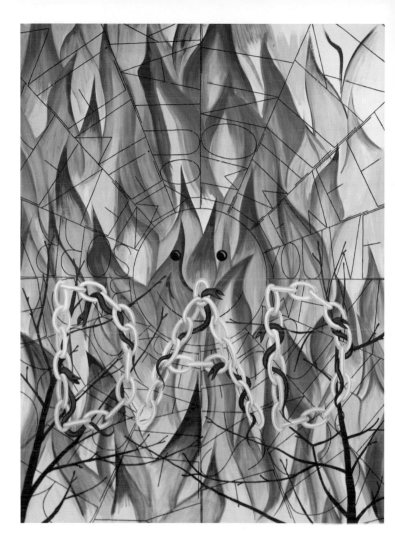

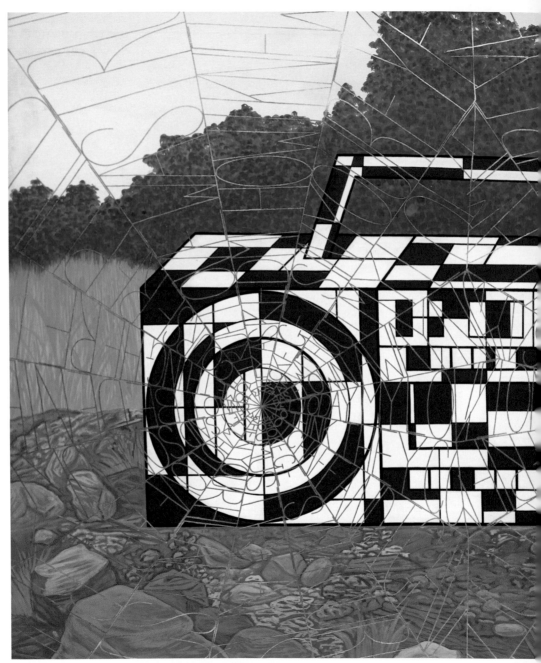

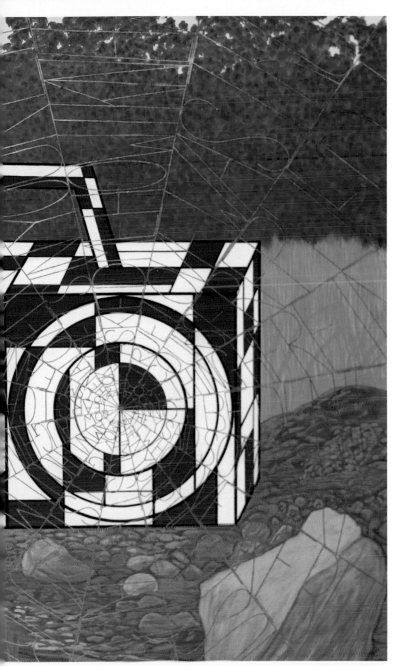

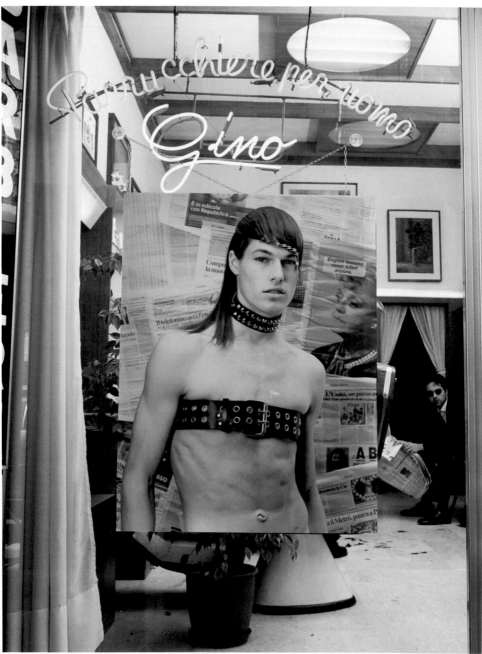

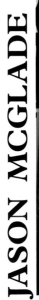

JASON MCGLADE

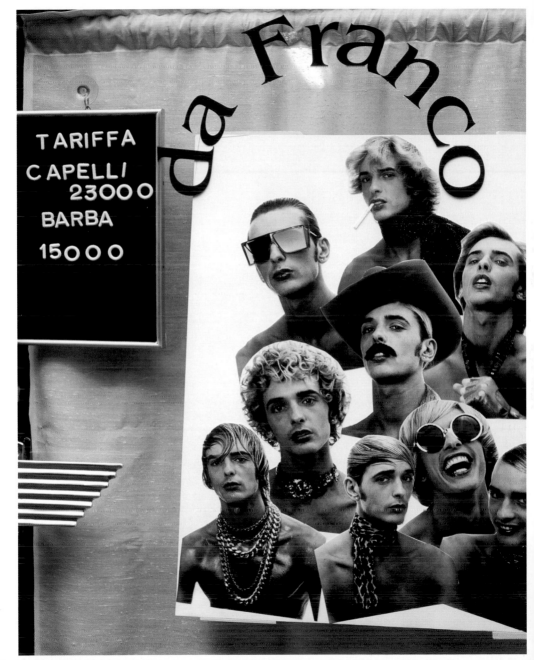

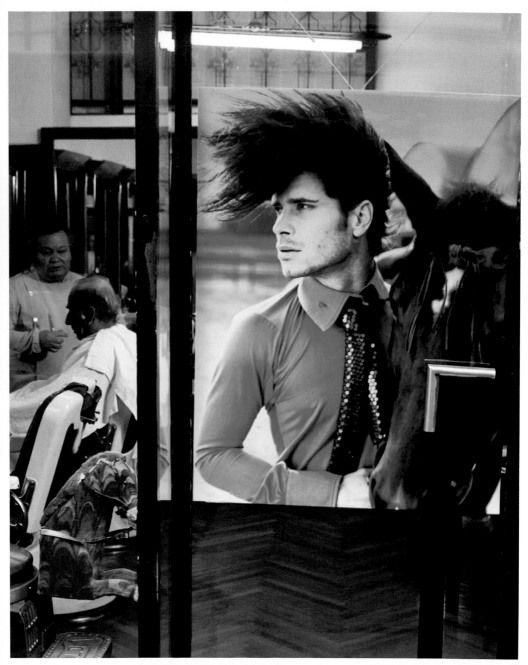

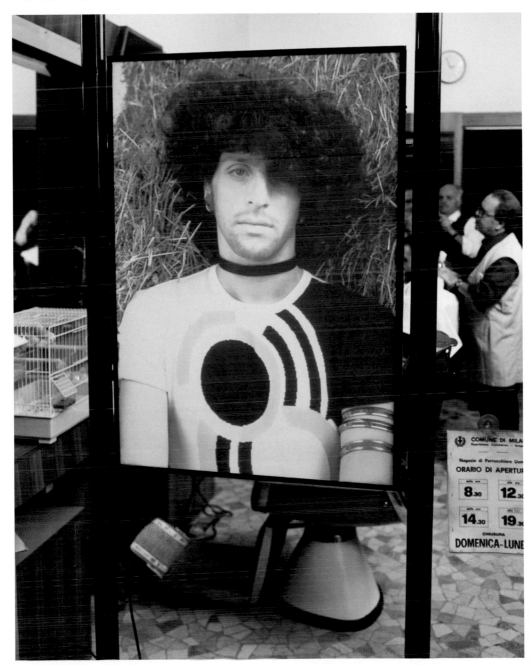

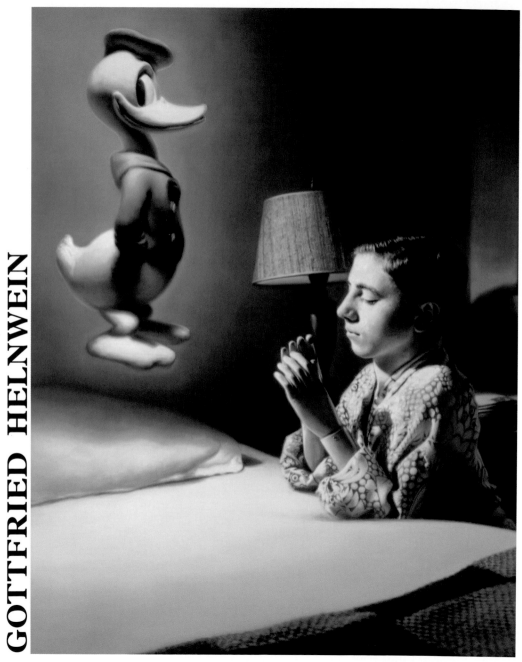

GOTTFRIED HELNWEIN

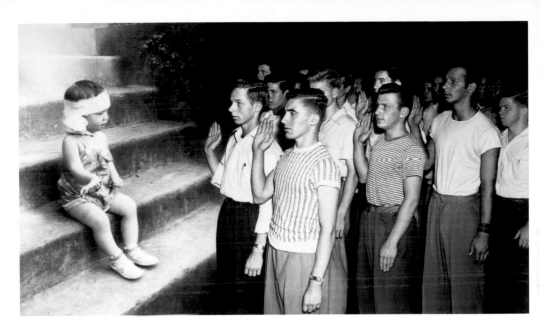

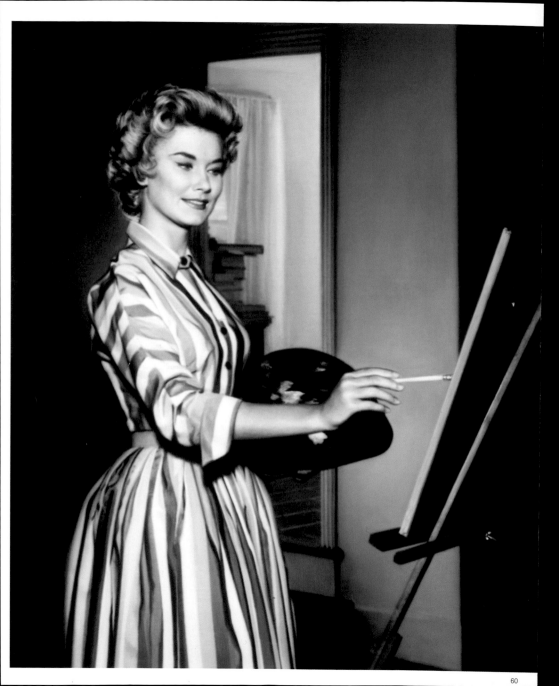

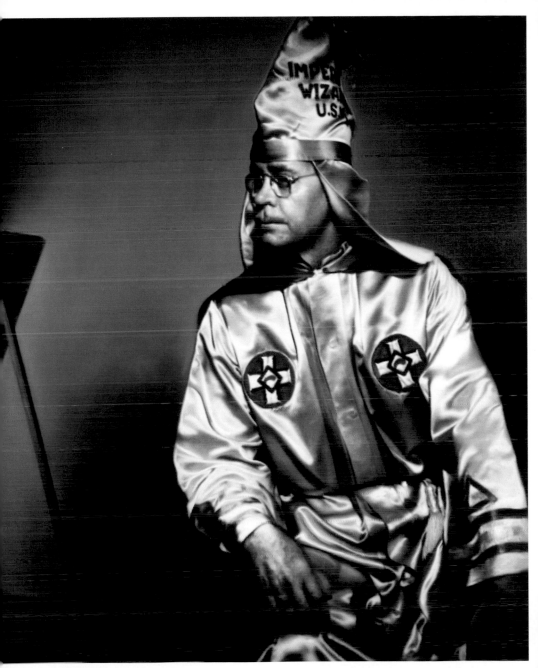

BOHDAN CAP

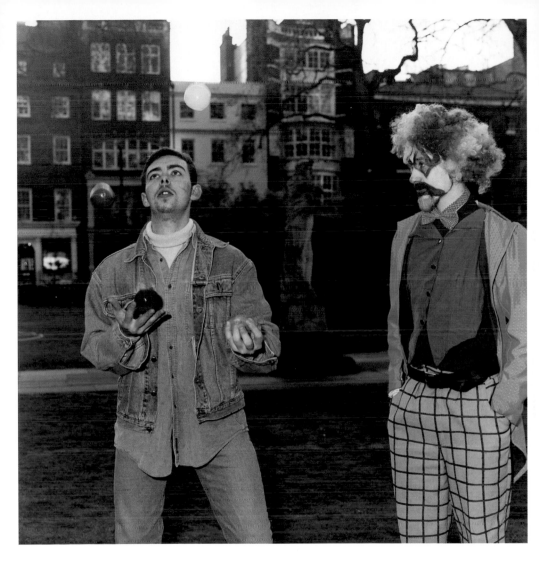

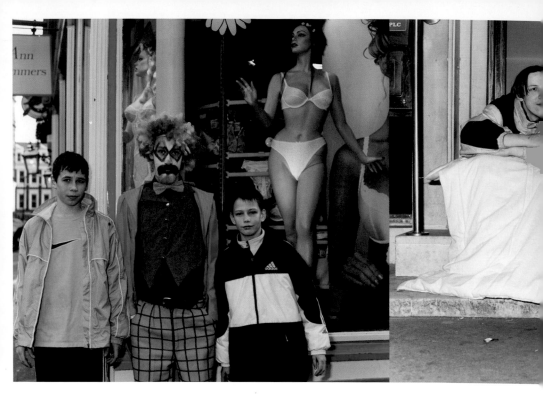

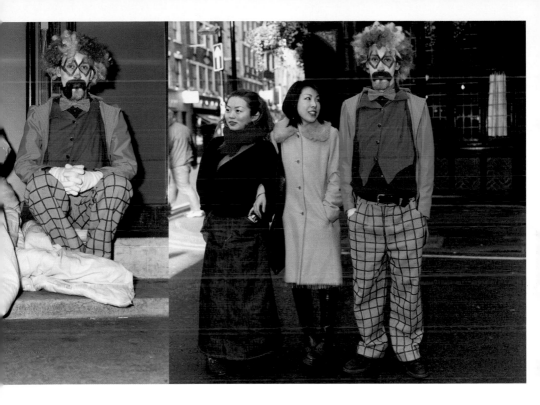

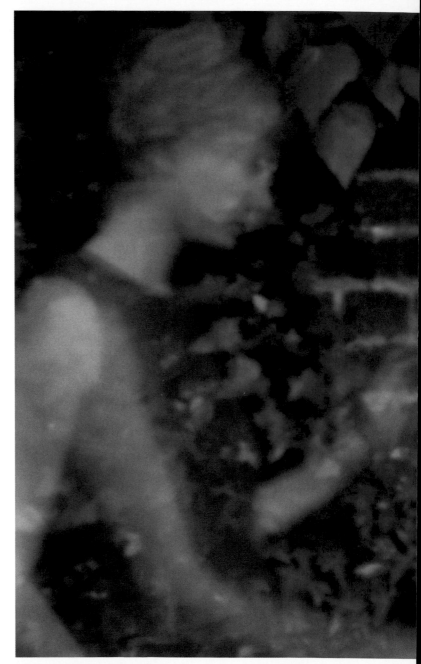

JAN DUNNING

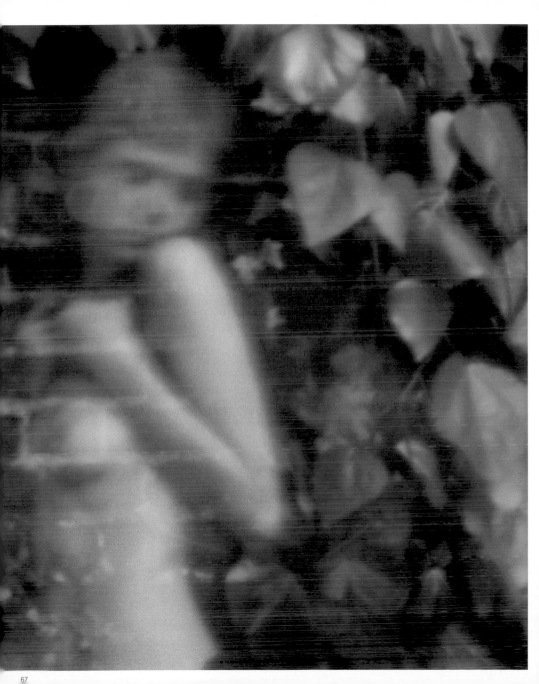

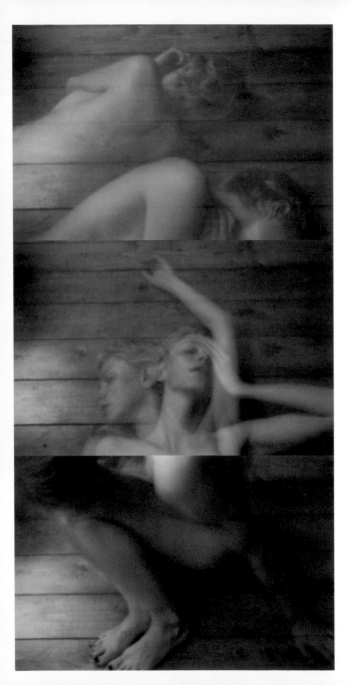

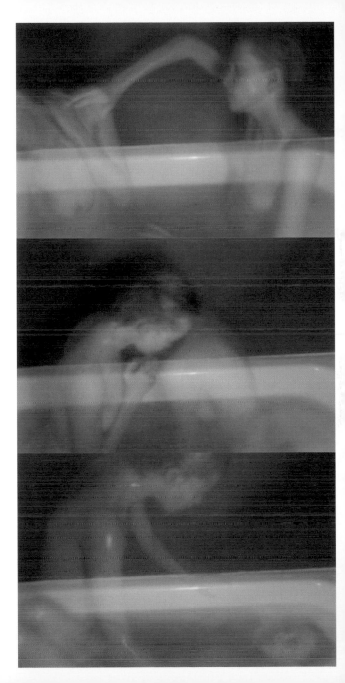

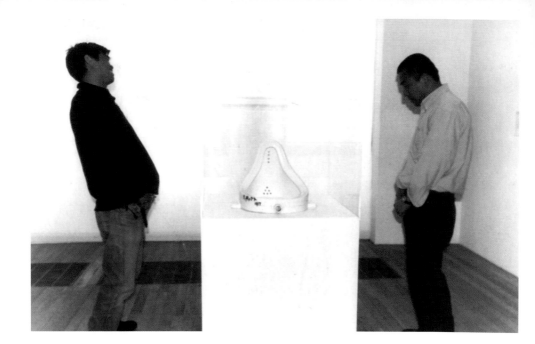

CAI YUAN & JJ XI

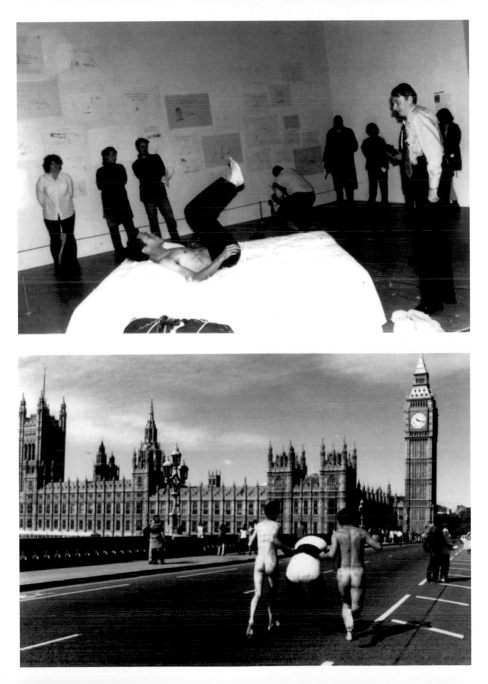

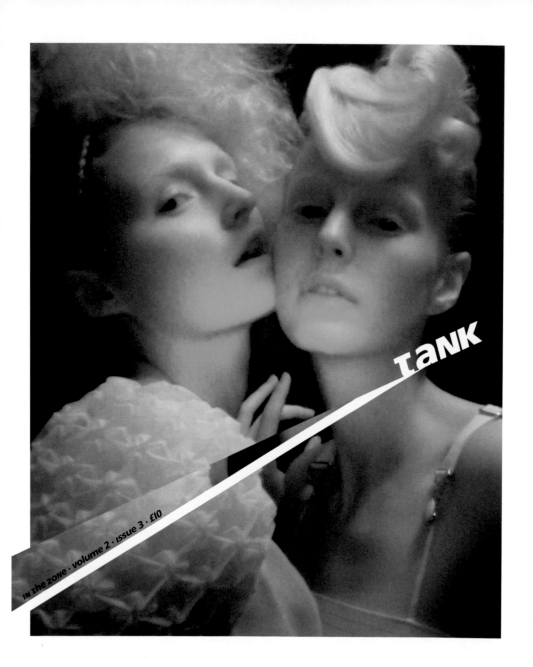

TANK

IN THE ZONE · volume 2 · issue 3 · £10

IN THE ZONE

VOLUME 2 · ISSUE 3 · MARCH 2001 · COVER PHOTOGRAPH BY MASOUD

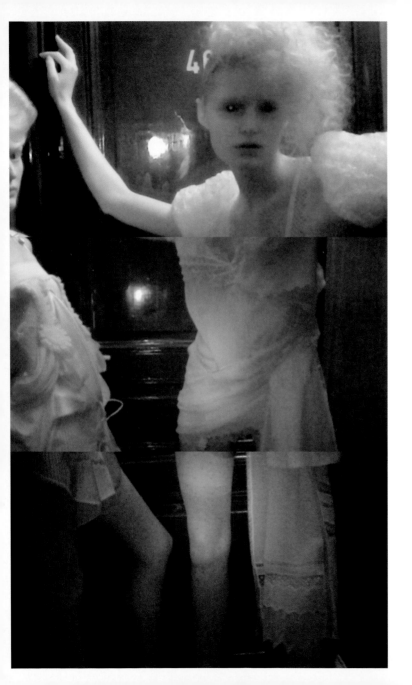

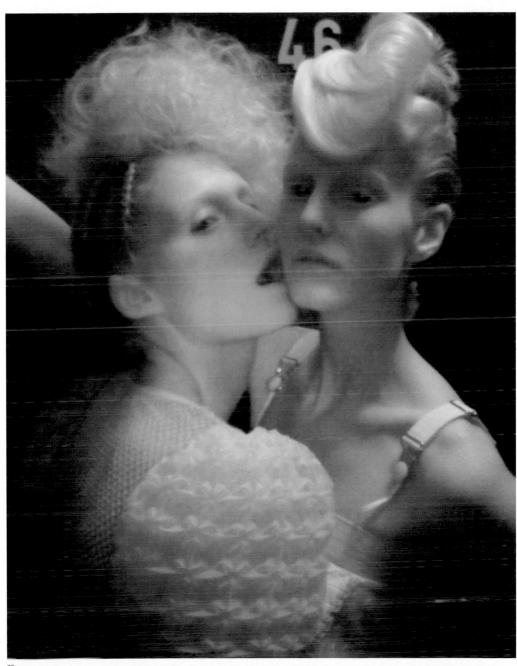

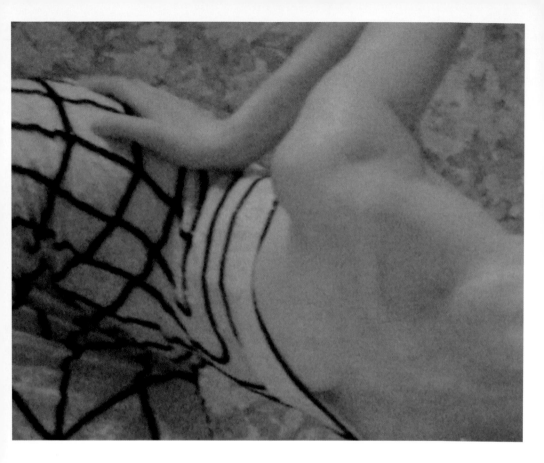

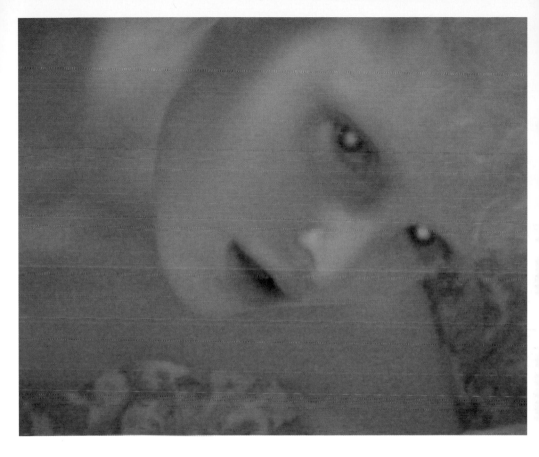

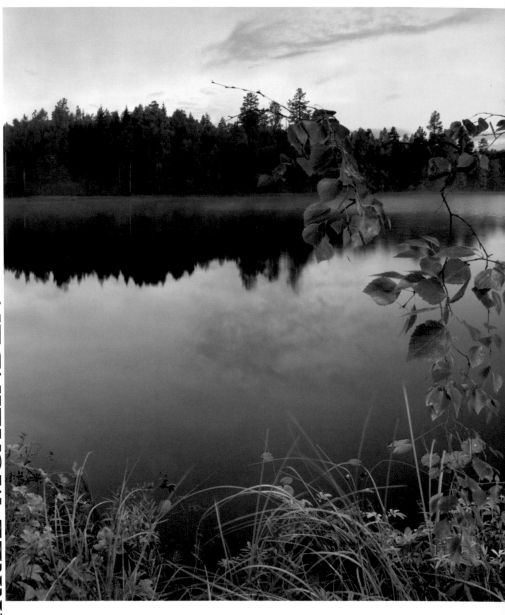

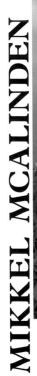

MIKKEL MCALINDEN

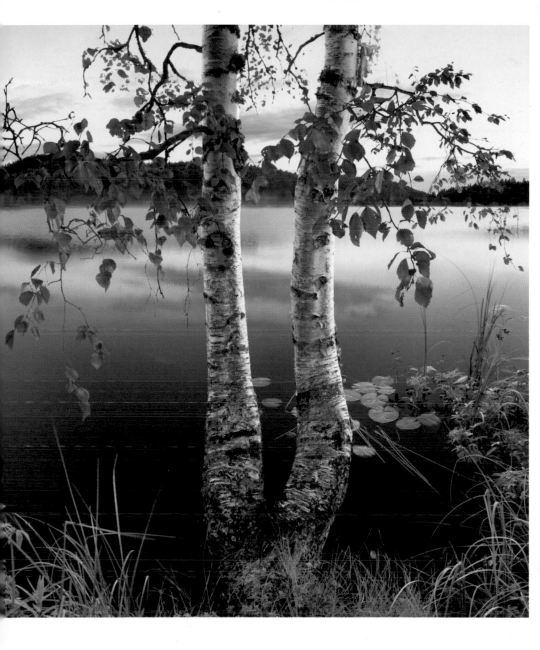

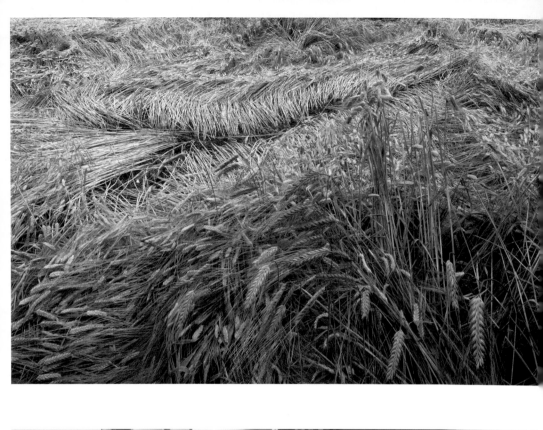

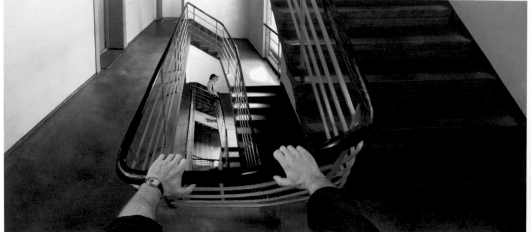

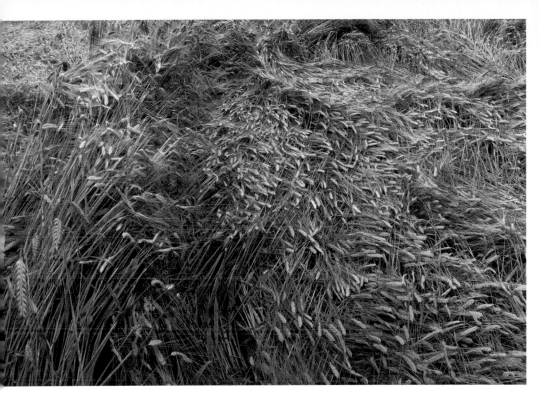

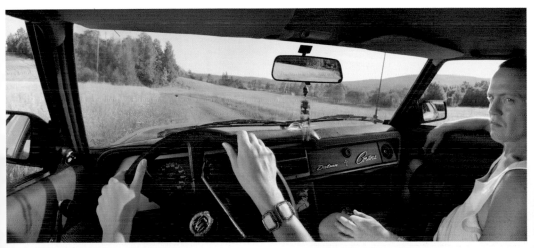

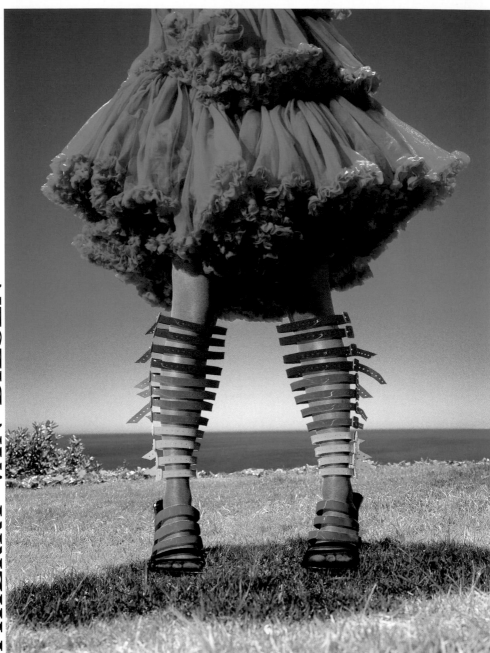

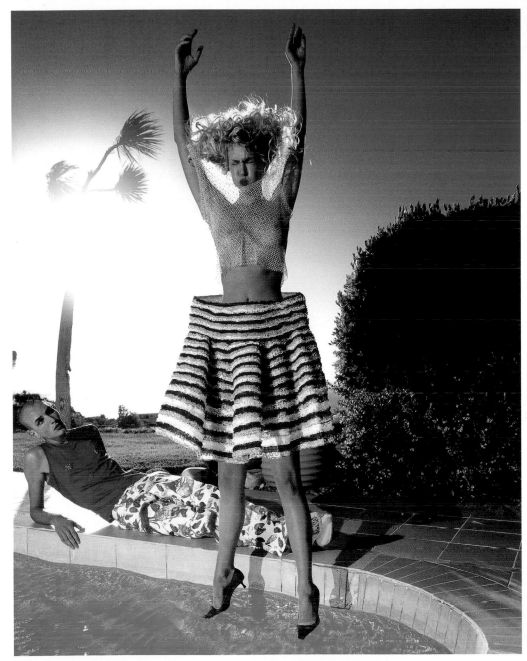

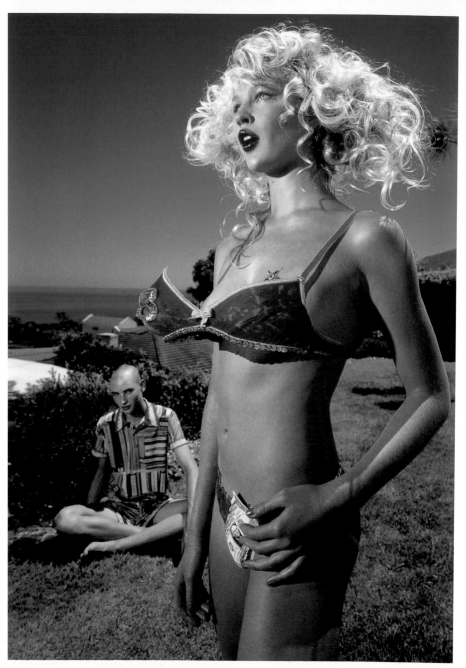

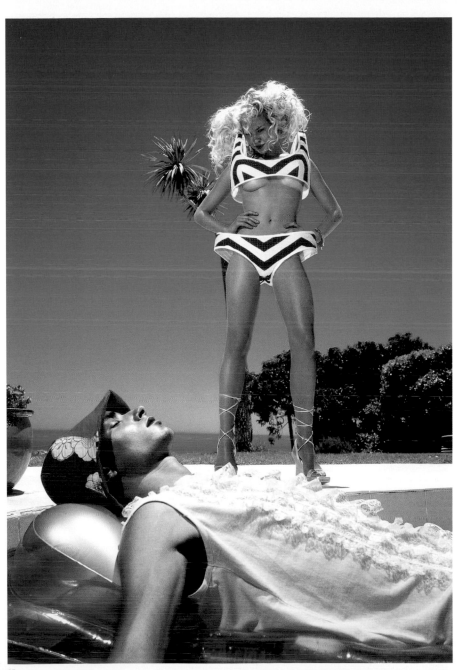

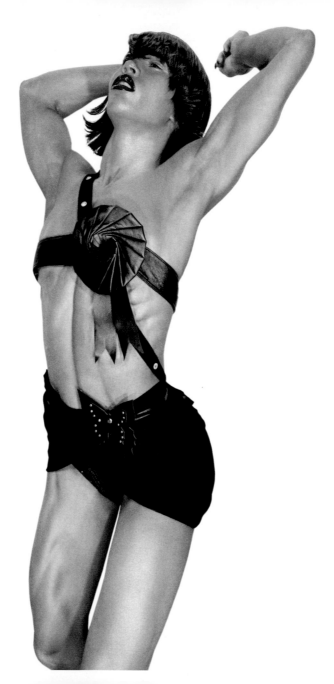

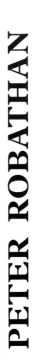

PETER ROBATHAN

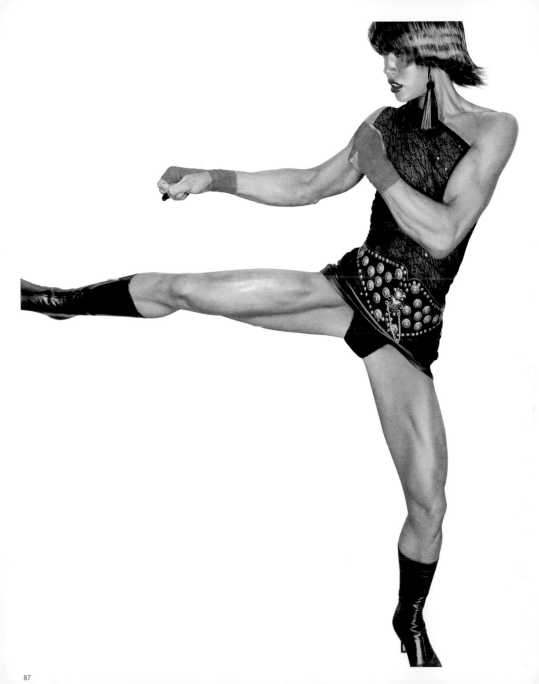

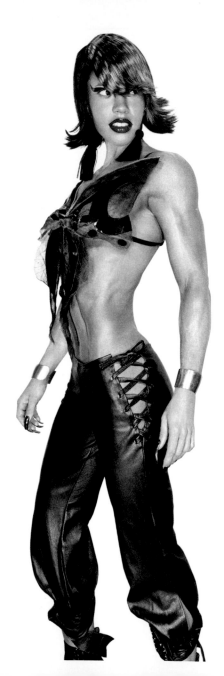

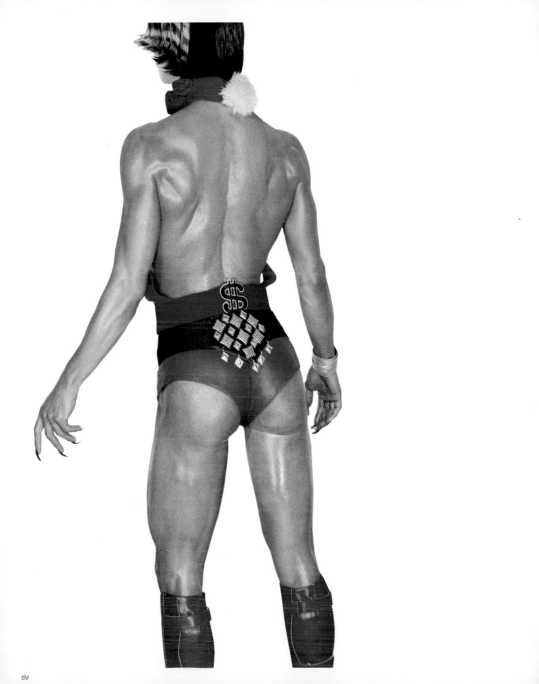

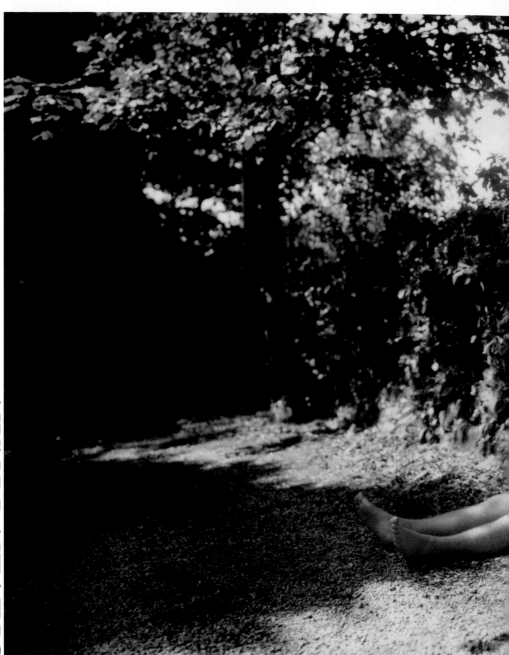

STEVEN TYNAN

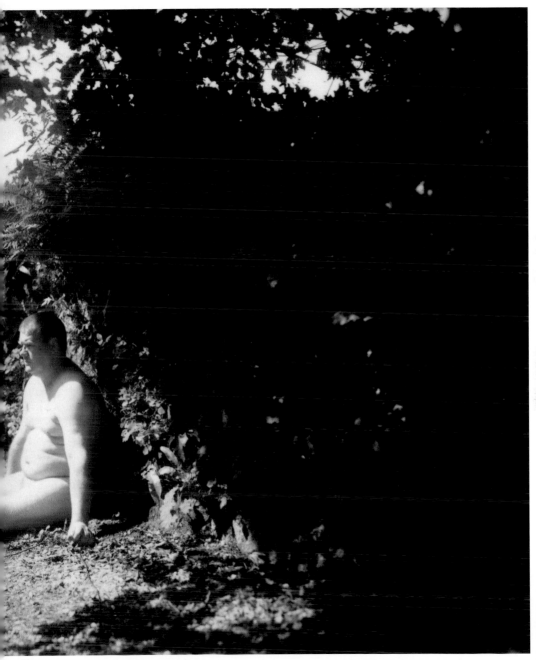

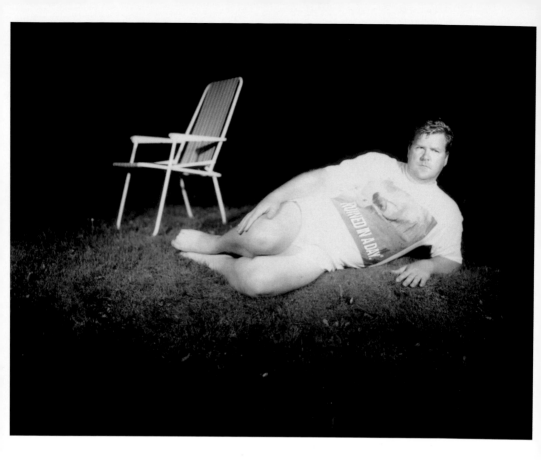

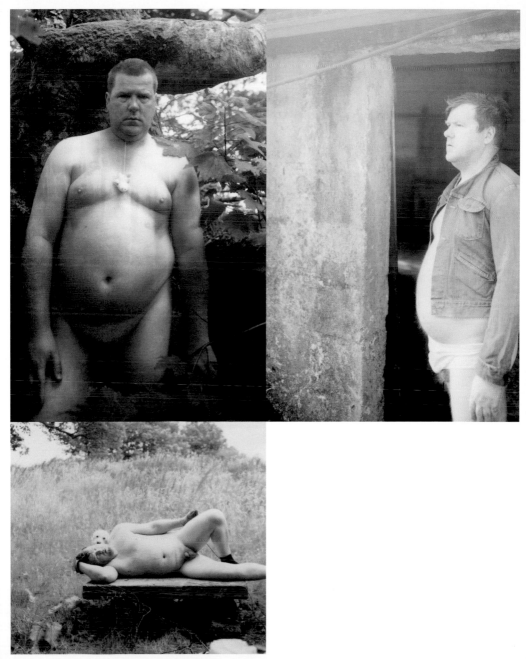

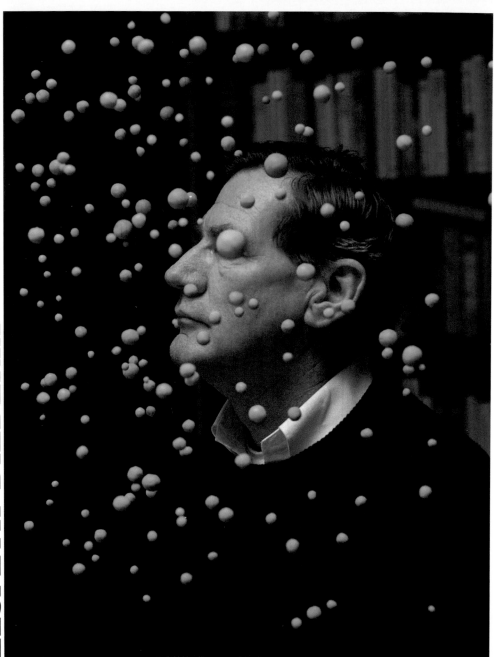

ELSPETH DIEDERIX

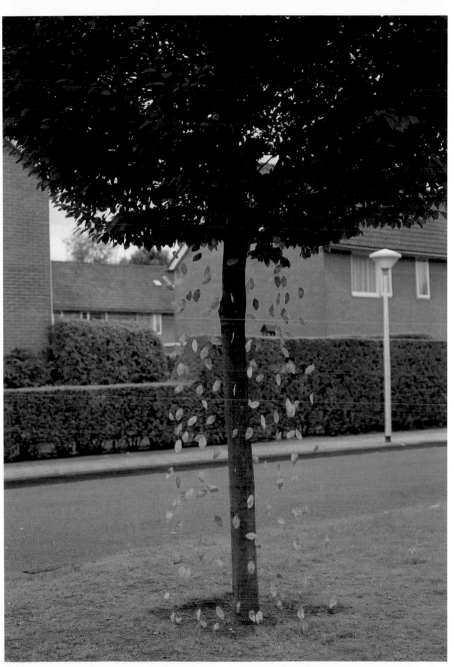

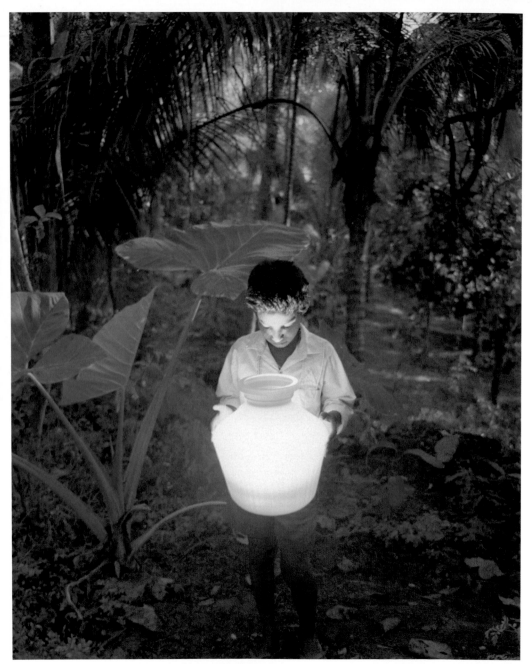

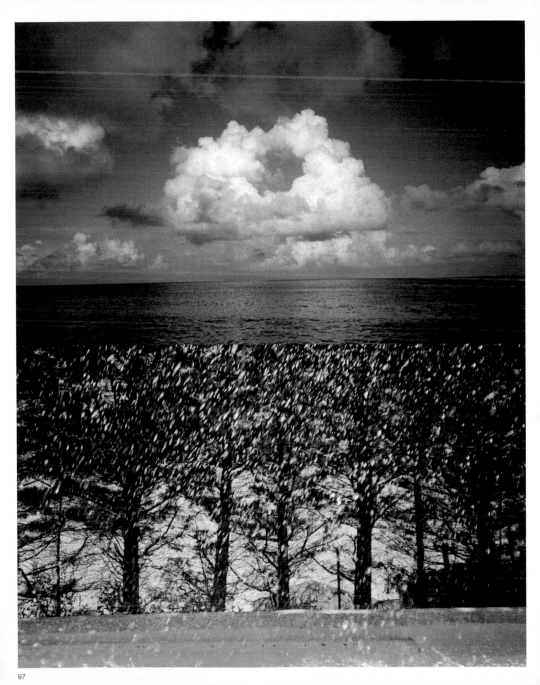

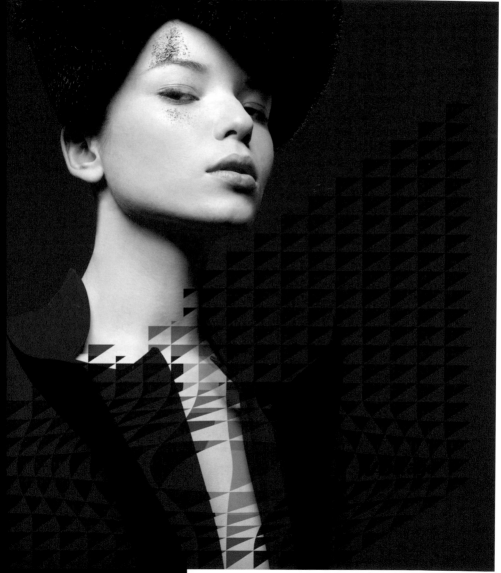

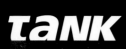

IGNITION FOR THE NATION

VOLUME 2 · ISSUE 4 · MAY 2001 · COVER PHOTOGRAPH BY MASOUD

Moorguards
18th. April 2001

Dear Julian
Here are the photos of our neighbours' cattle.
They did not have foot and mouth disease but
were considered a dangerous contact.

The beasts were piled up, yards from the
house where five children live.
After two days we could smell the stench from ½ mile away.
The shiny blob on the right bottom corner is a calf
expelled by the bloated carcass of it's mother.
Two of the bullocks they couldn't catch so they
chased them round the field taking pop shots
with rifles at them.

After 8 days MAFF said that they suspected that
one or two of the cattle were over 5 years old so
could they please be sorted into age groups, and
by the way, we would like the ear tags. Bruce said:
"Do it yourself"

Their sheep were herded into pens so violently that
they were dropping their lambs as they ran.
Some sheep have been herded into pens, shot, then
the next lot herded in on top of them and so on
until the pen is full.
Six days later animals have been found alive in heaps.

THIS IS OUR WORLD

love mum.

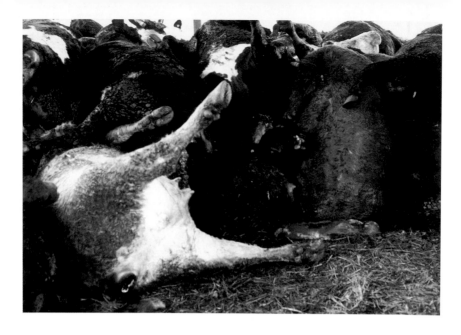

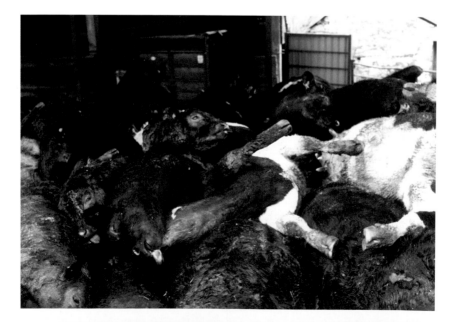

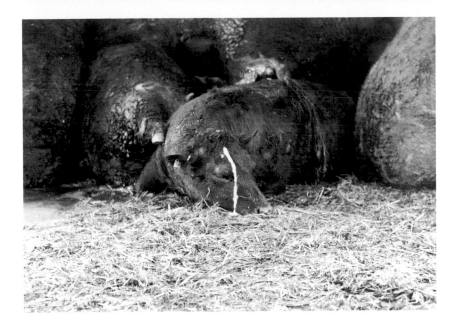

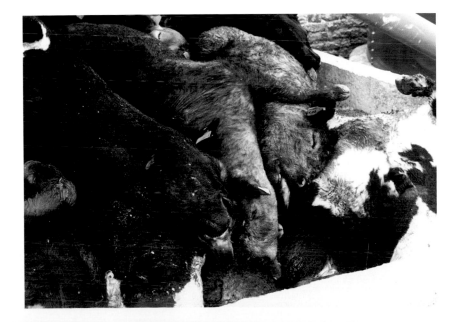

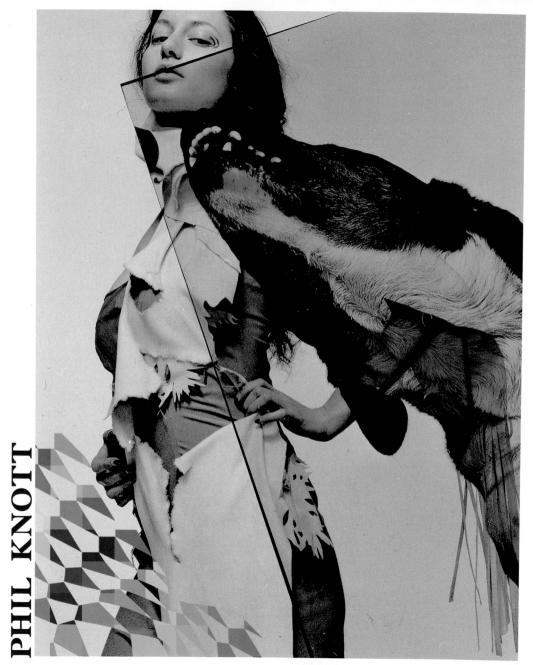

PHIL KNOTT

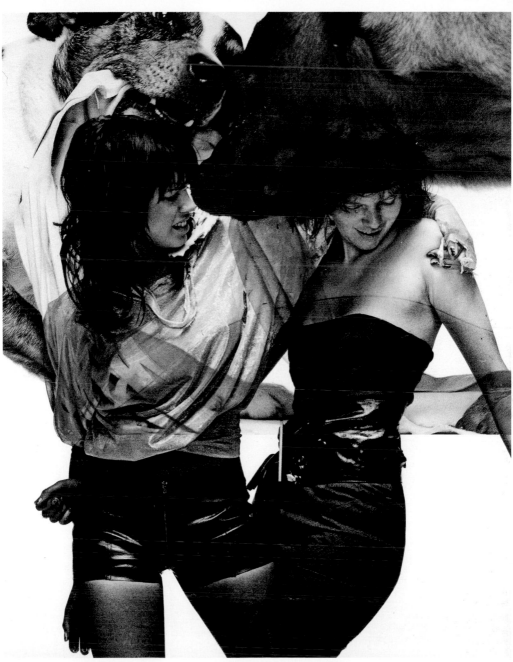

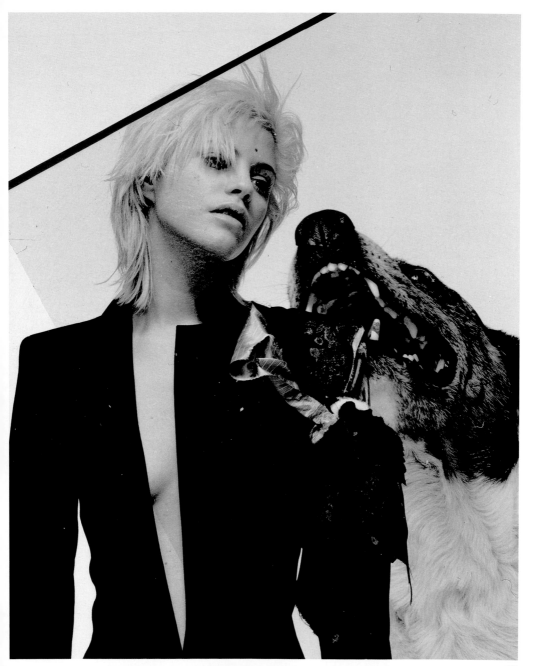

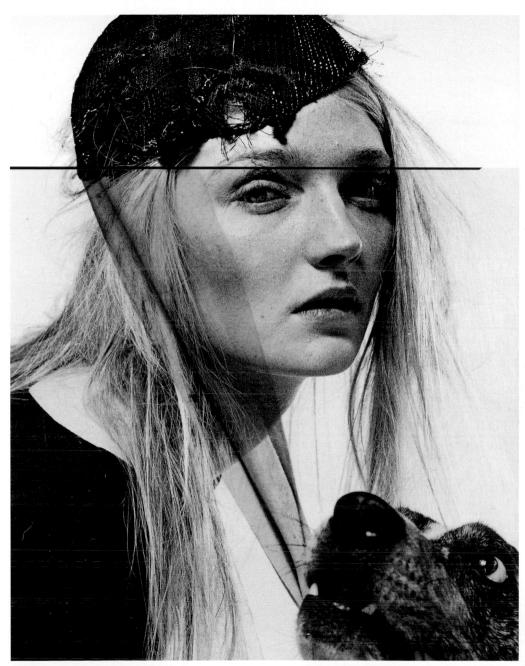

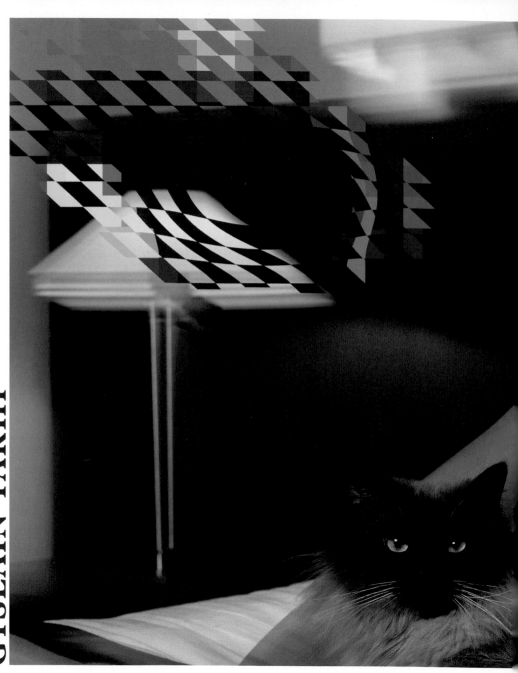

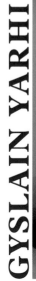

GYSLAIN YARHI

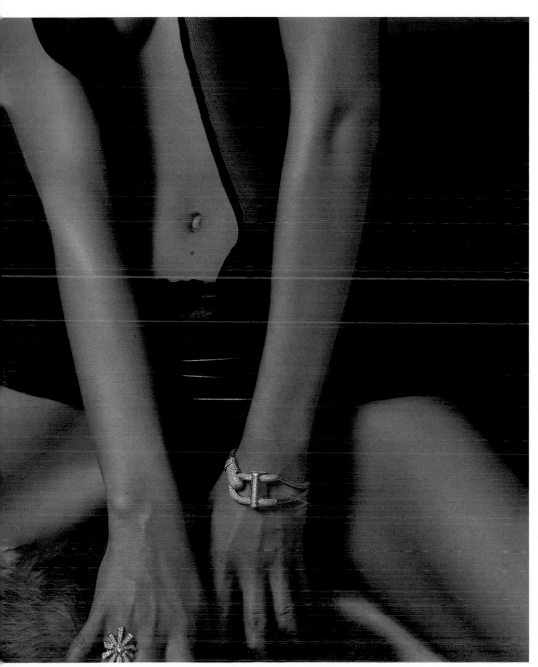

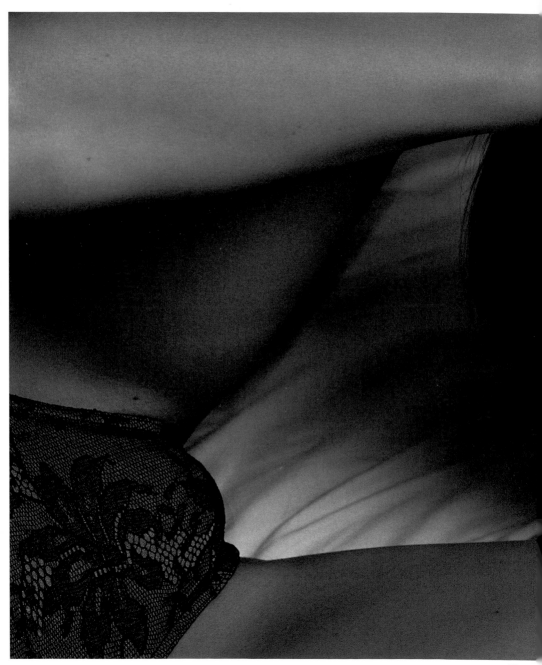

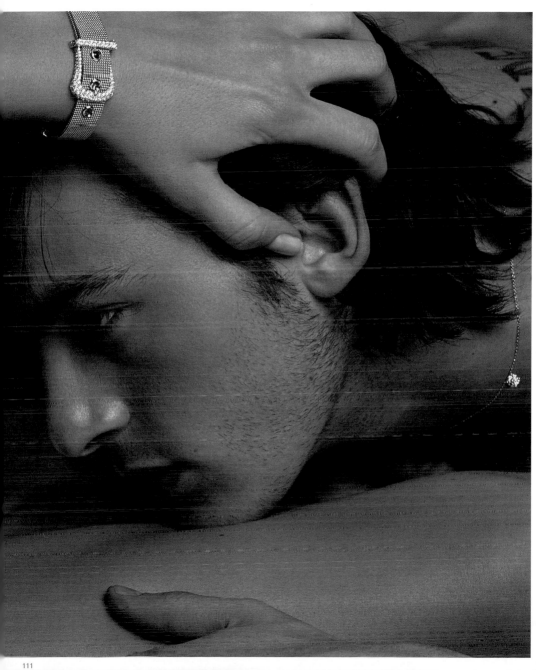

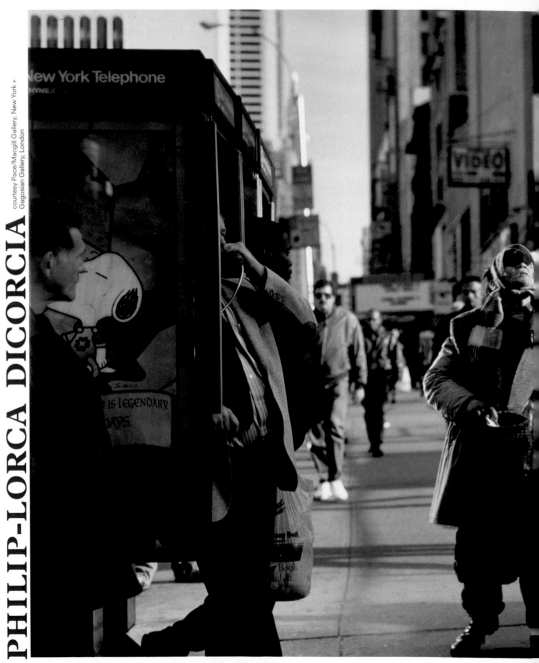

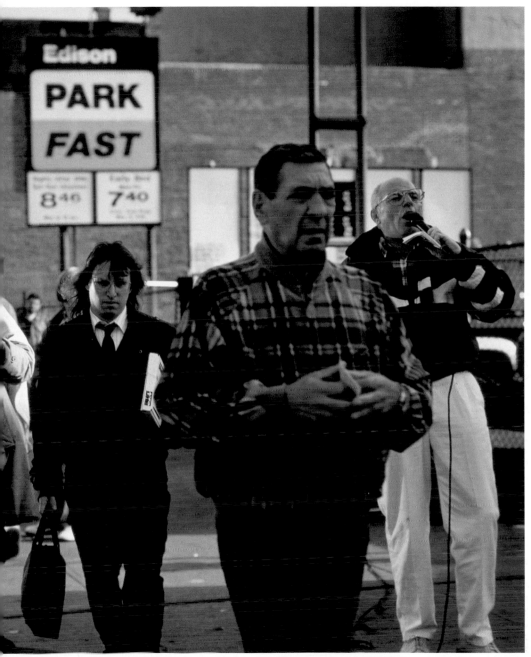

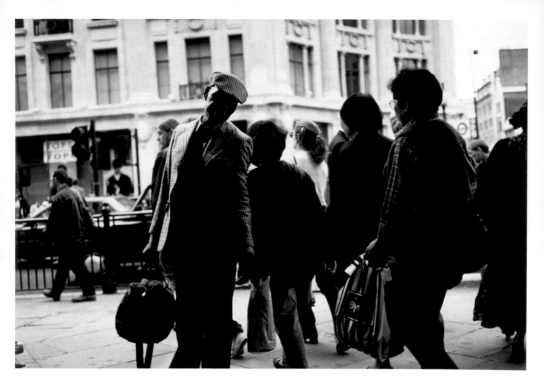

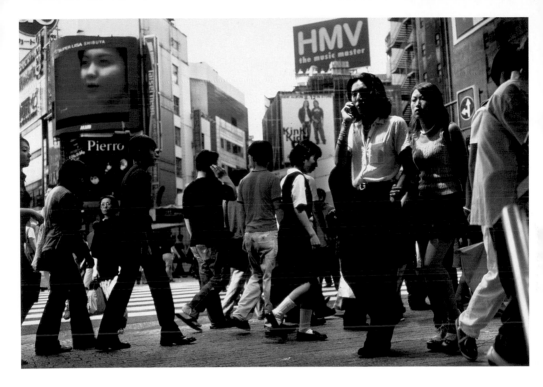

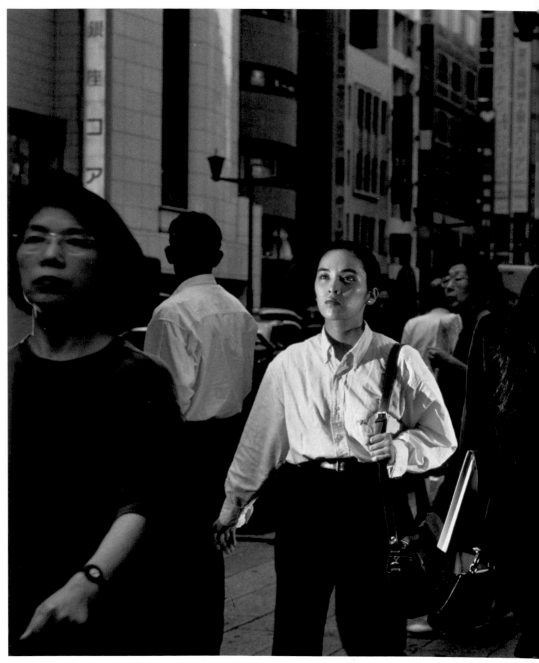

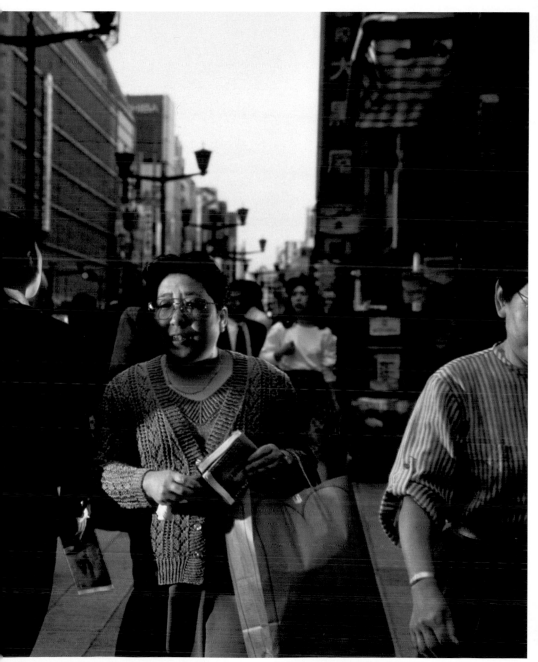

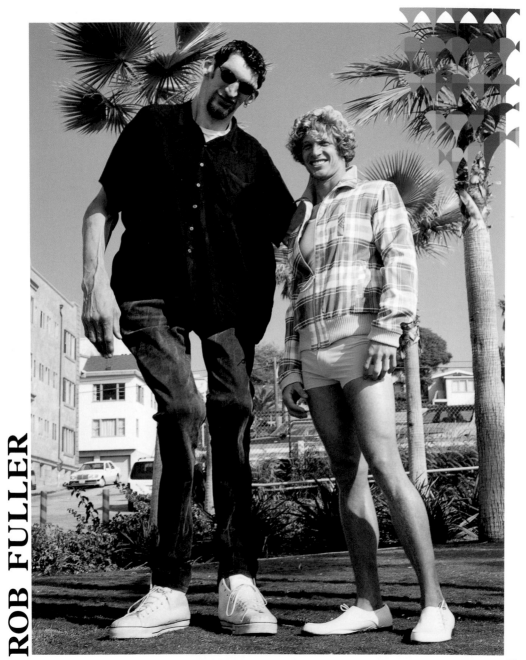

ROB FULLER

118

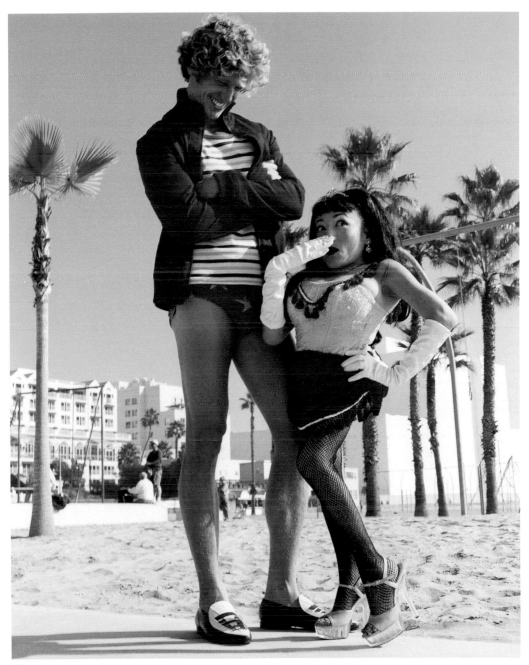

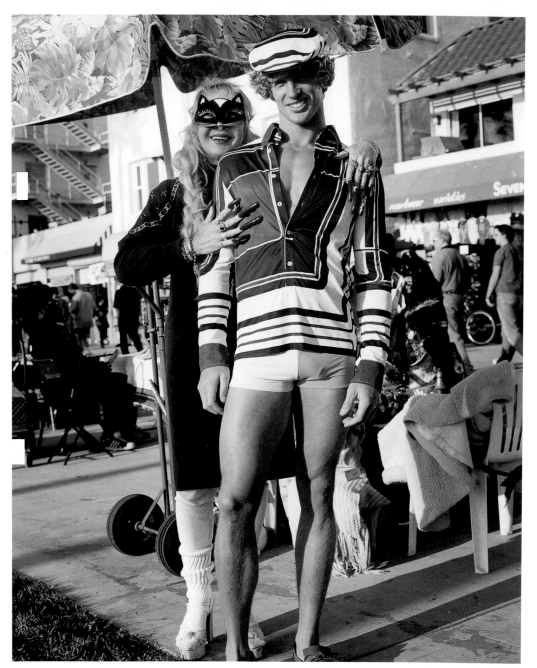

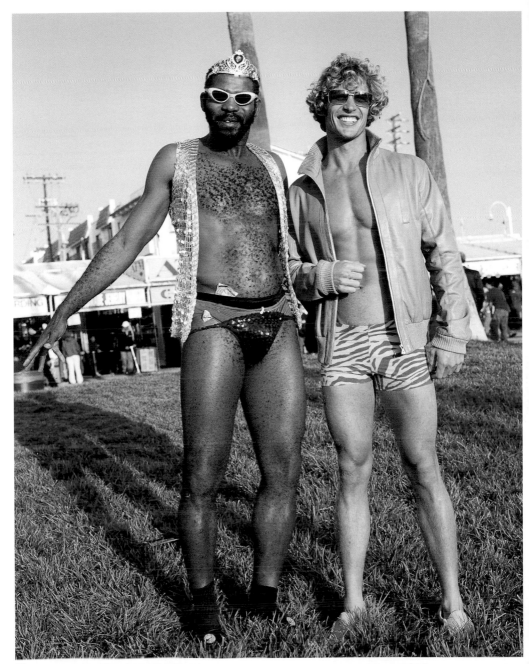

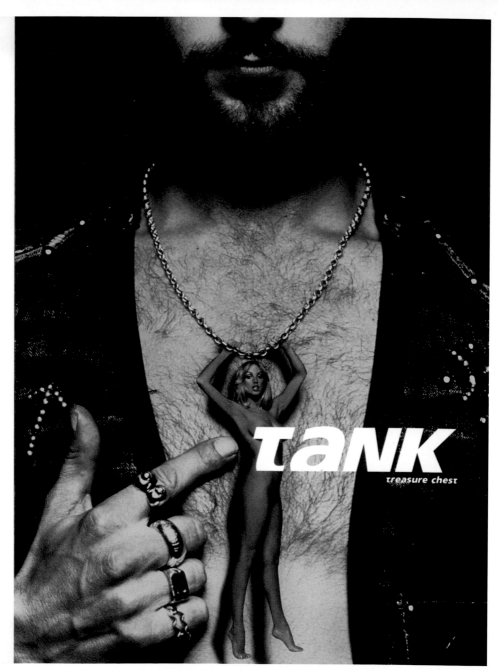

BIG DADDY

VOLUME 2 · ISSUE 5 · AUGUST 2001 · COVER ILLUSTRATION BY PETER BARRY

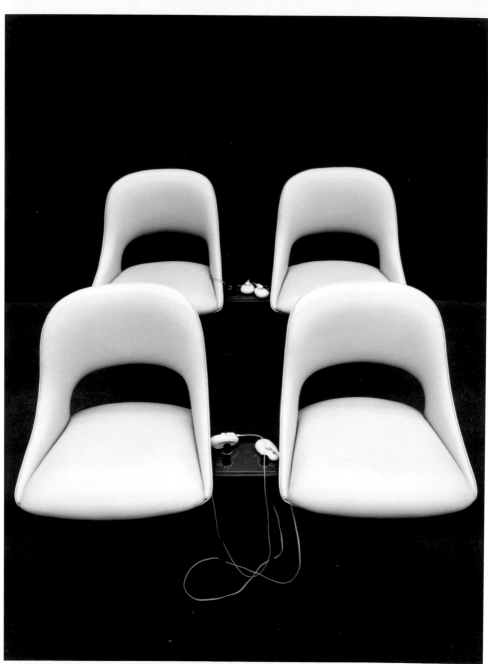

JASON ODDY

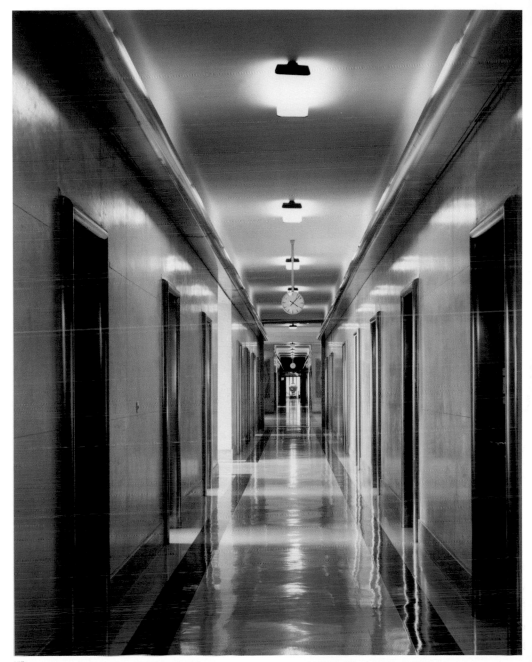

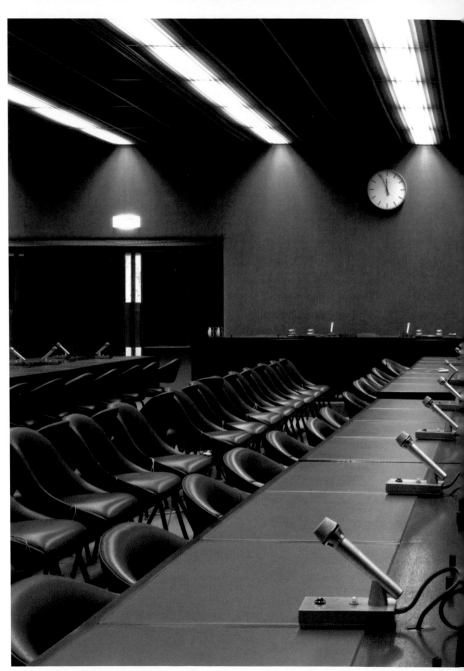

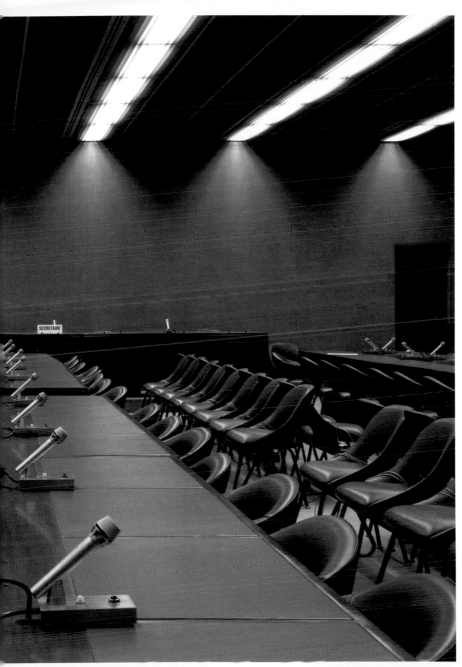

SECRETAIRE

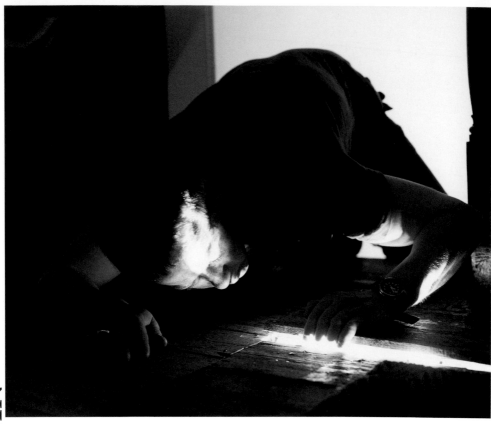

JULIAN BURGIN

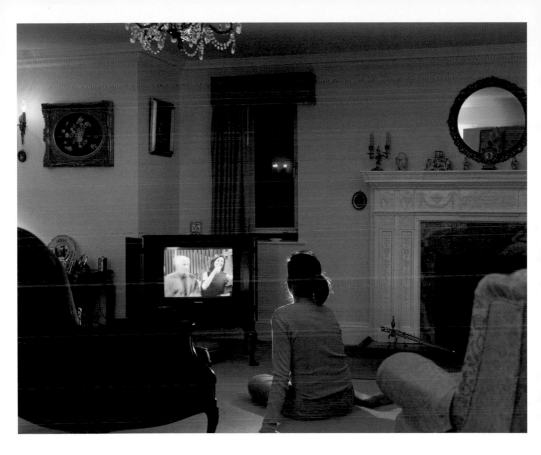

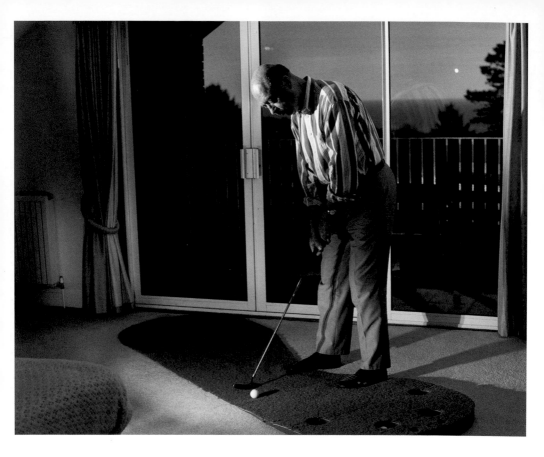

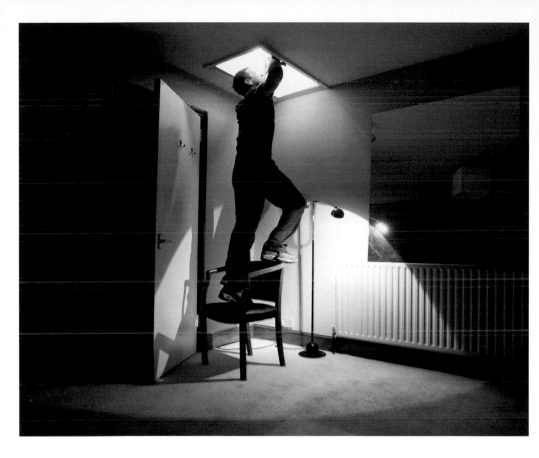

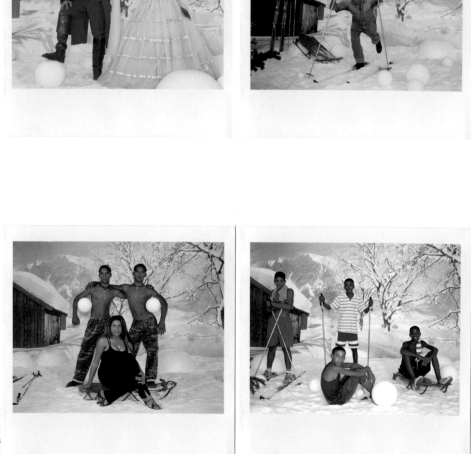

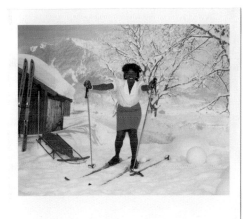

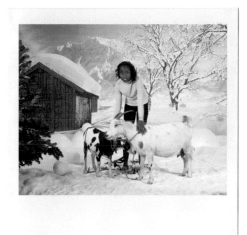

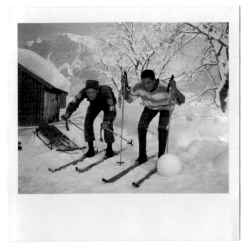

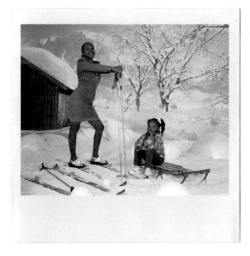

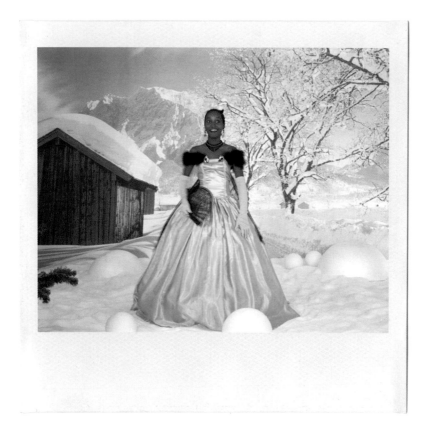

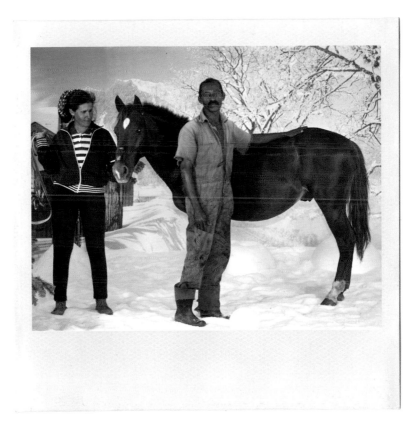

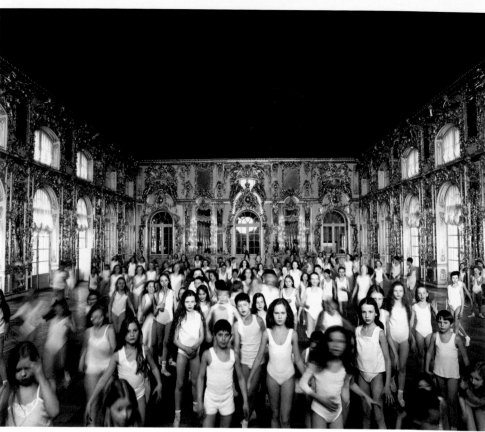

AES+F GROUP

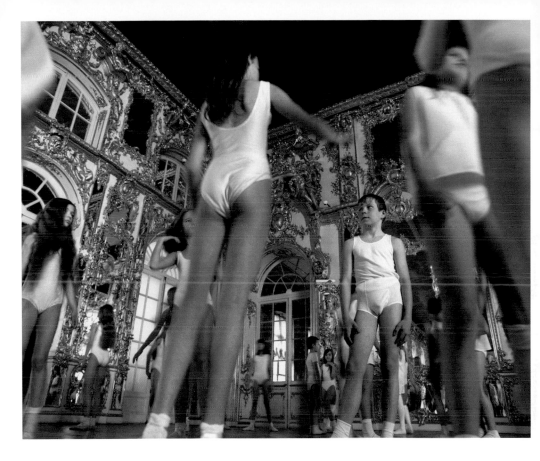

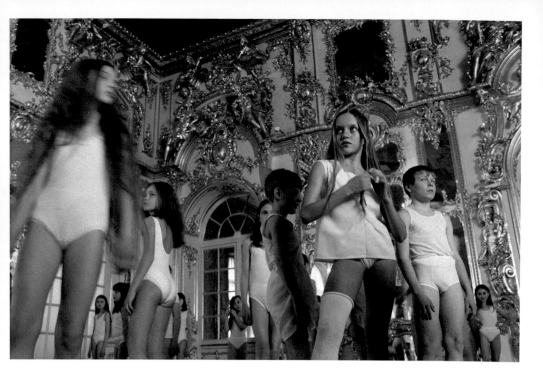

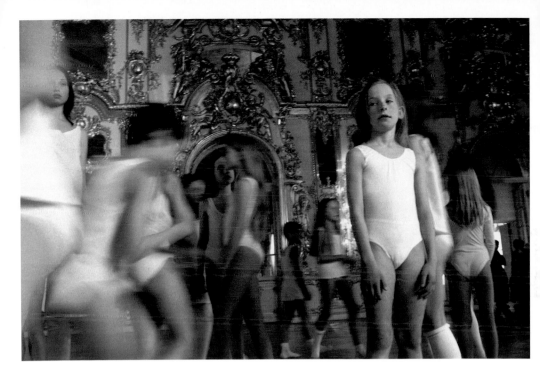

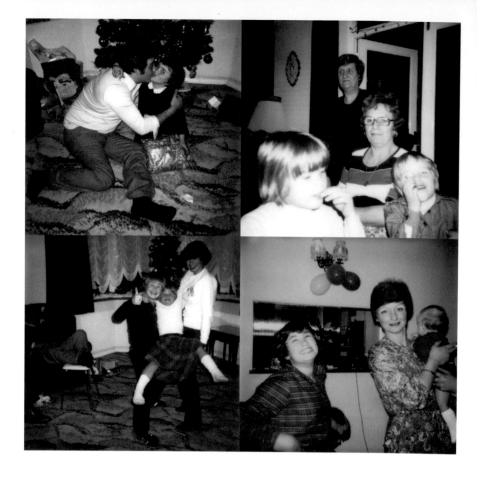

VICTORIA WOOLHEAD

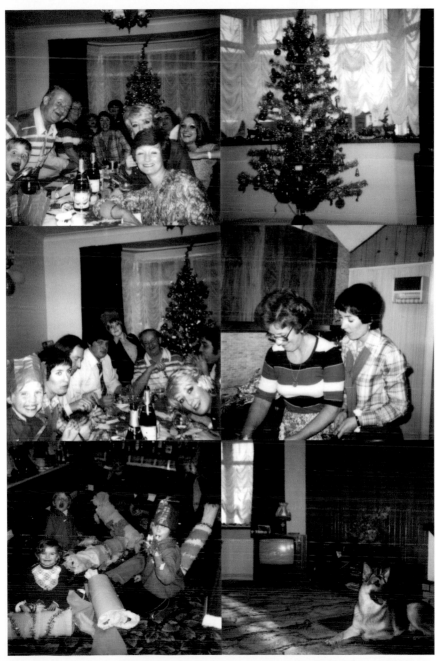

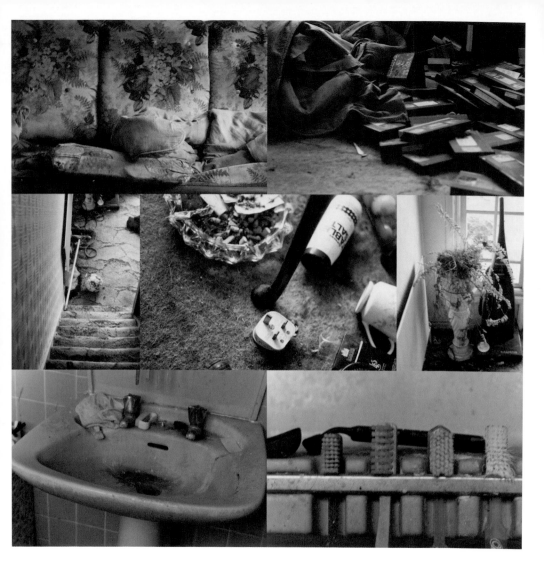

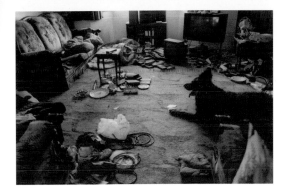

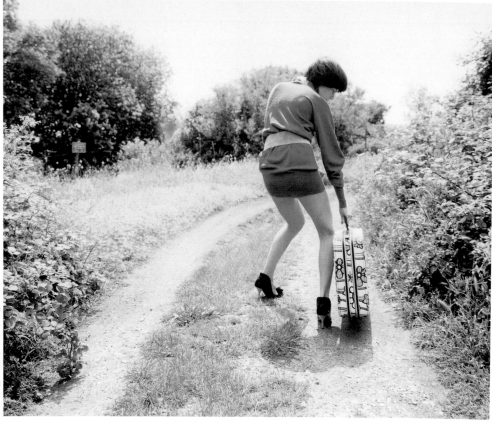

ANDREA SPOTORNO

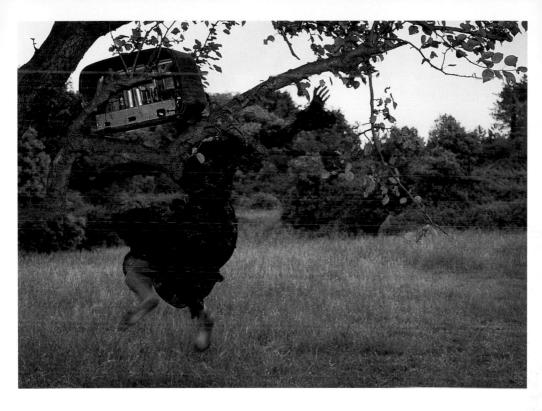

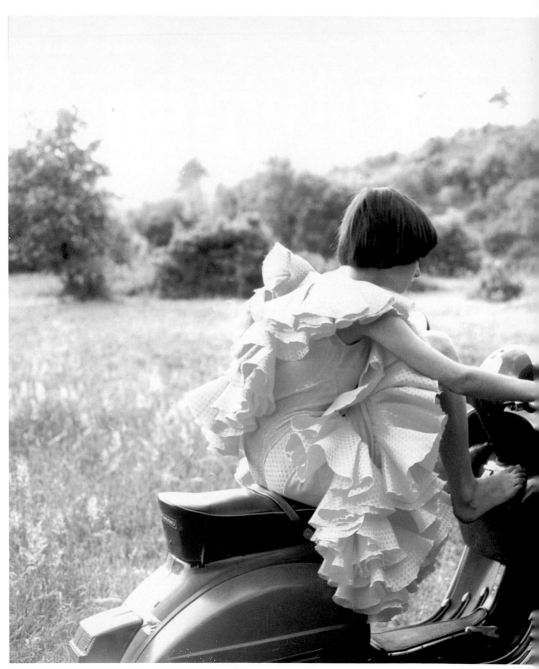

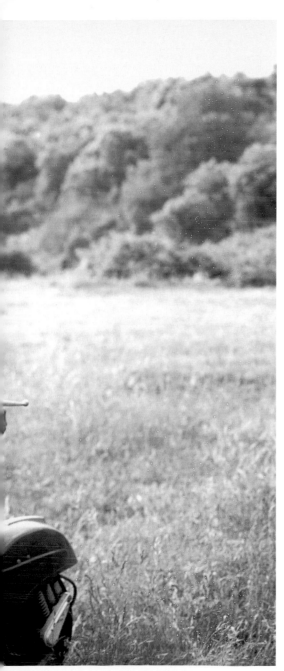

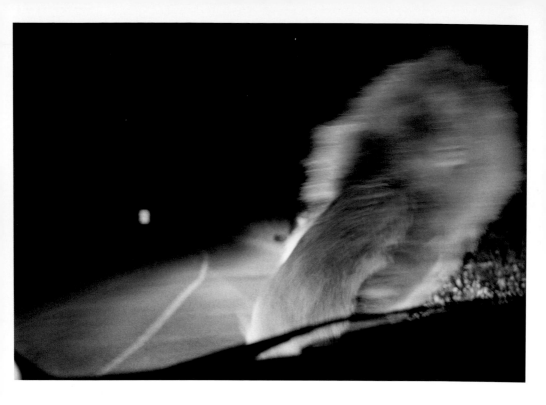

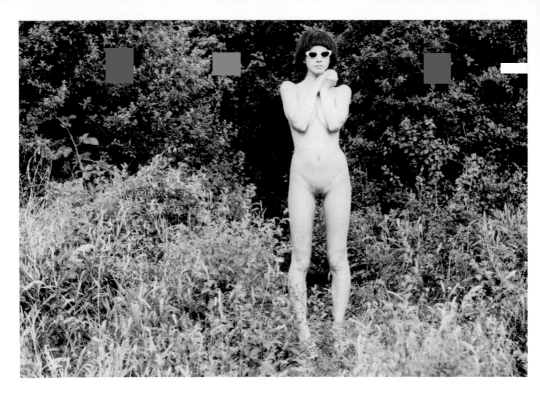

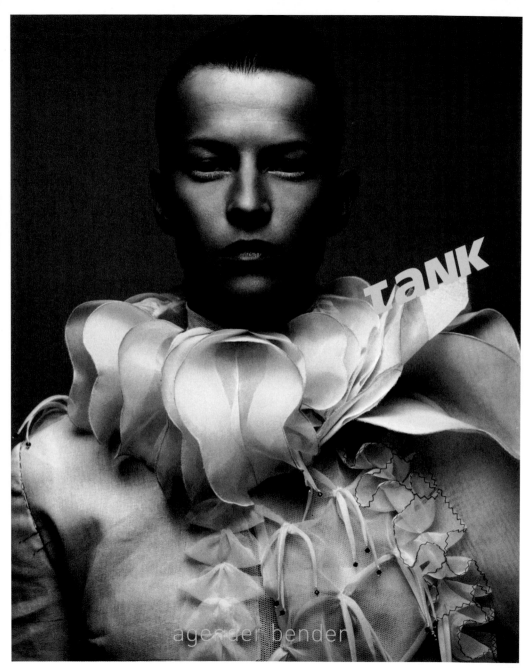

TANK

agender bender

HARD AND FAST RULES

VOLUME 2 · ISSUE 6 · OCTOBER 2001 · COVER PHOTOGRAPH BY GREG LOTUS

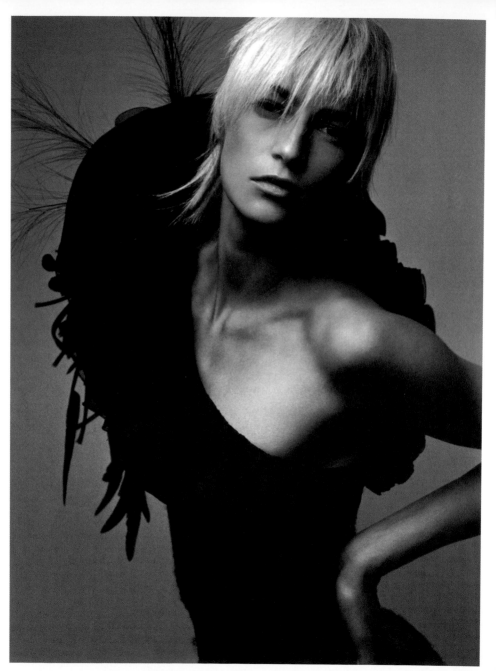

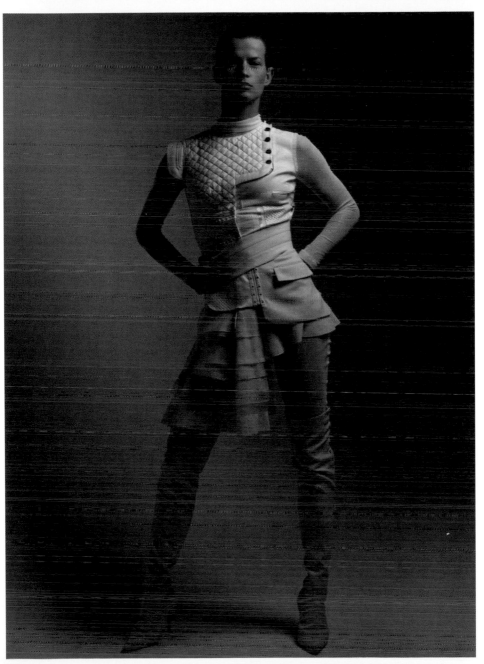

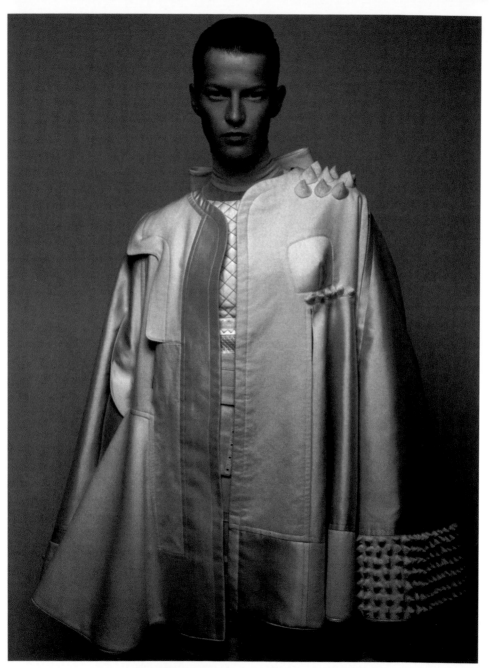

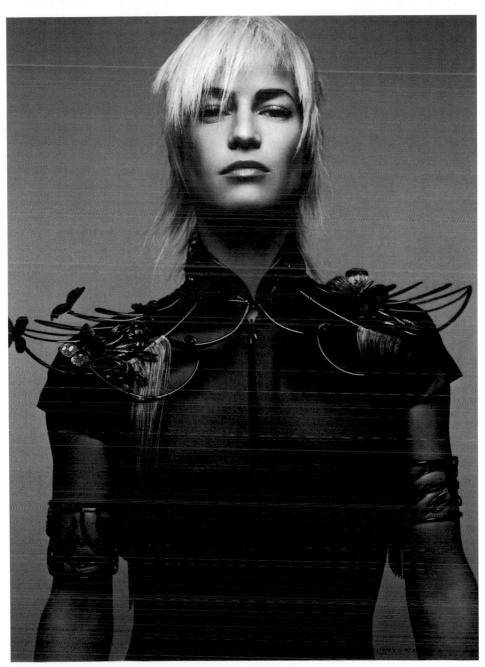

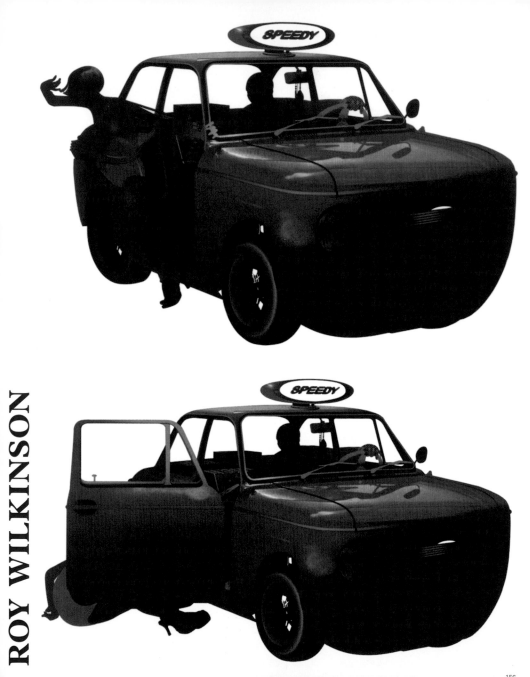

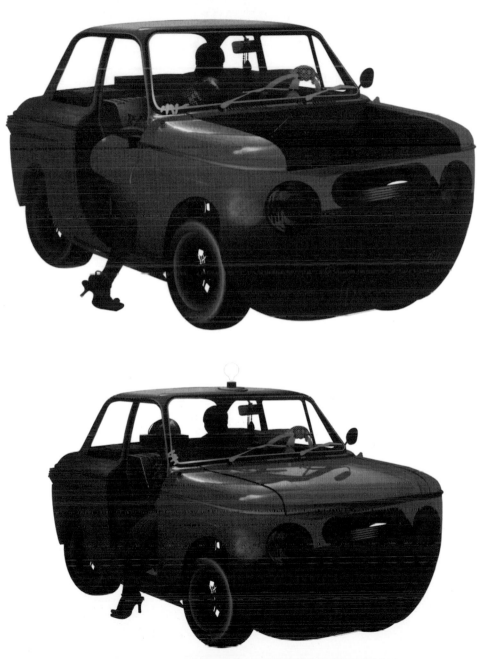

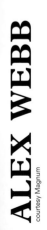

ALEX WEBB

courtesy Magnum

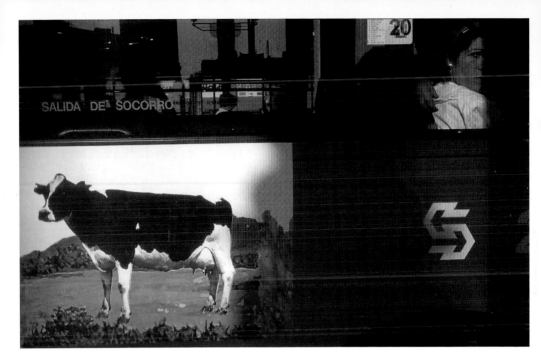

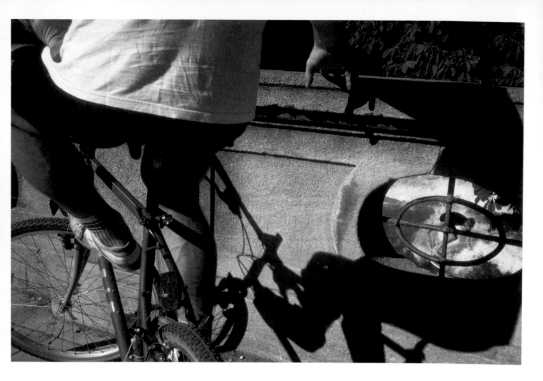

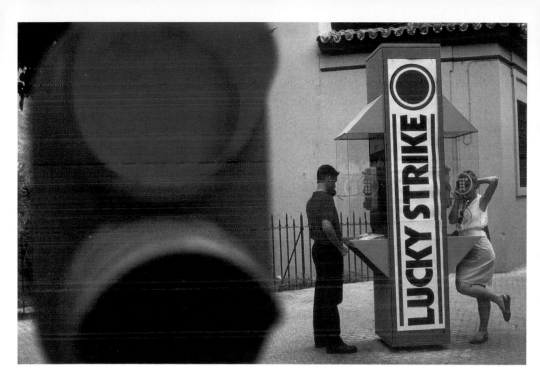

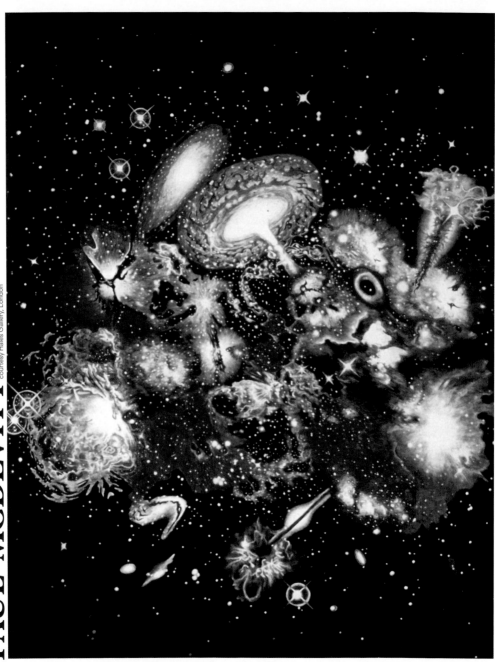

162

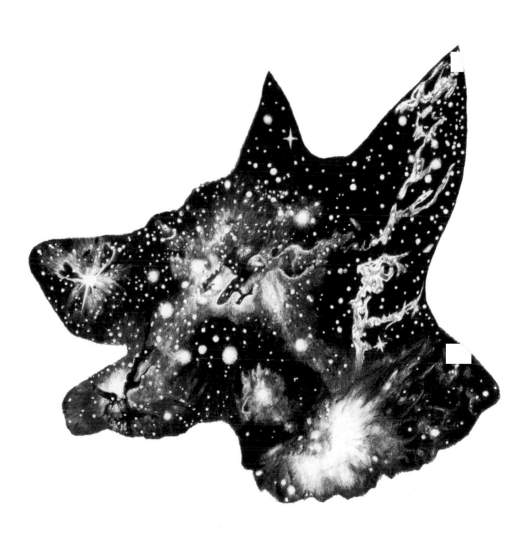

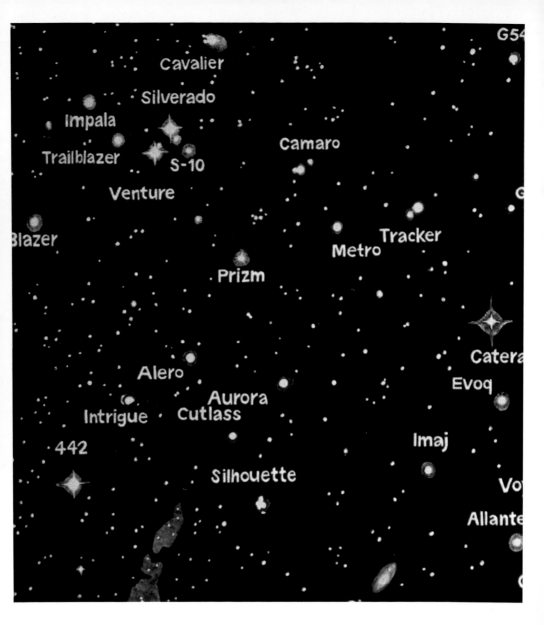

G54

Cavalier

Silverado

Impala

Camaro

Trailblazer

S-10

Venture

Blazer

Tracker

Metro

Prizm

Catera

Alero

Evoq

Intrigue   Aurora
            Cutlass

442

Imaj

Silhouette

Vo

Allante

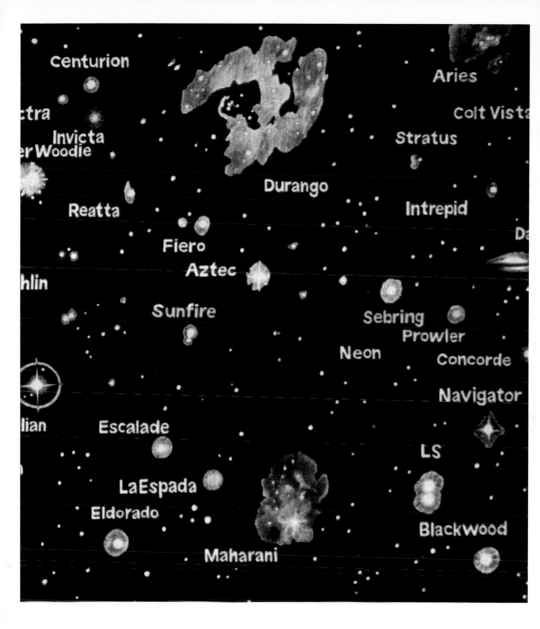

ALEXANDRA KINGA FEKETE

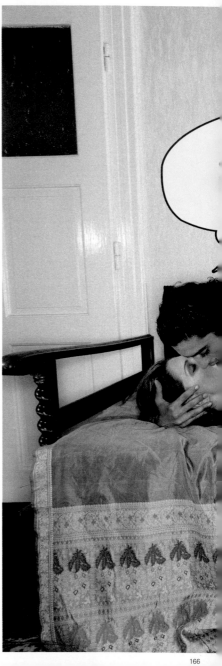

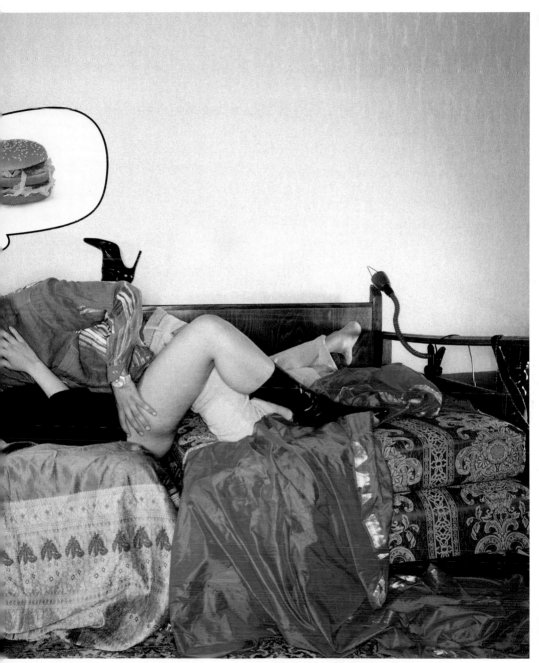

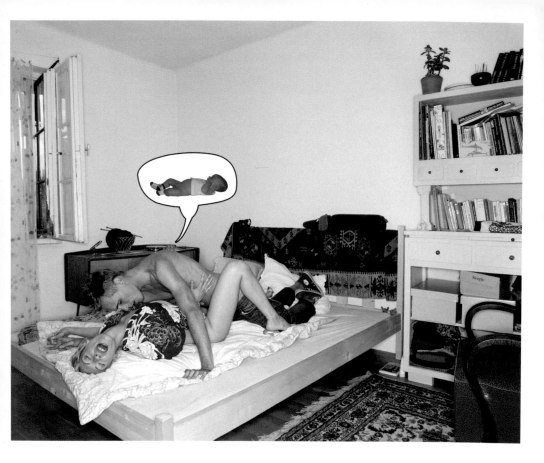

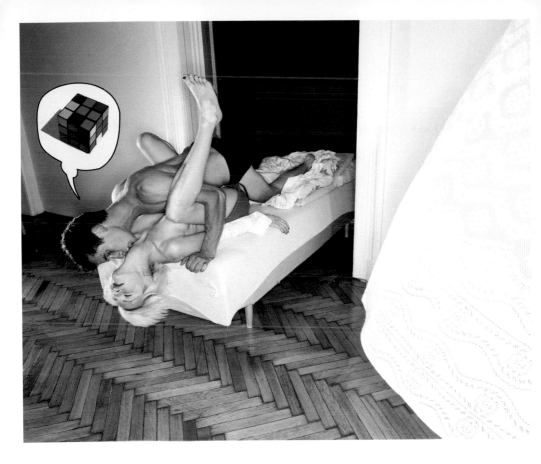

SPENCER TRACE + STACEY WILLIAMS

embroidery by Debbie Stack + Jennifer Carr

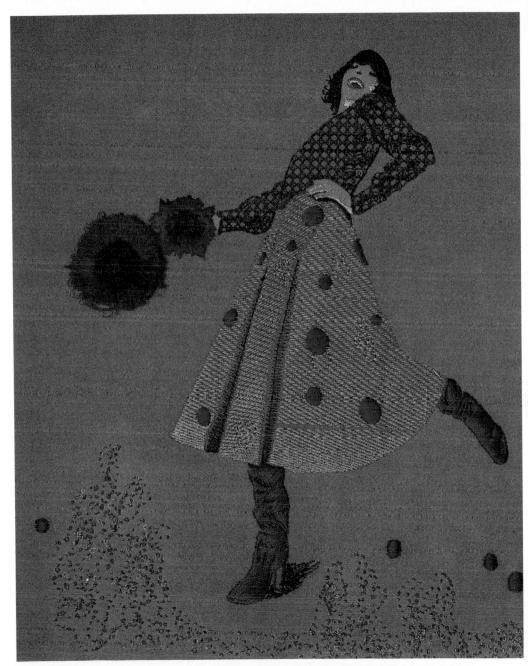

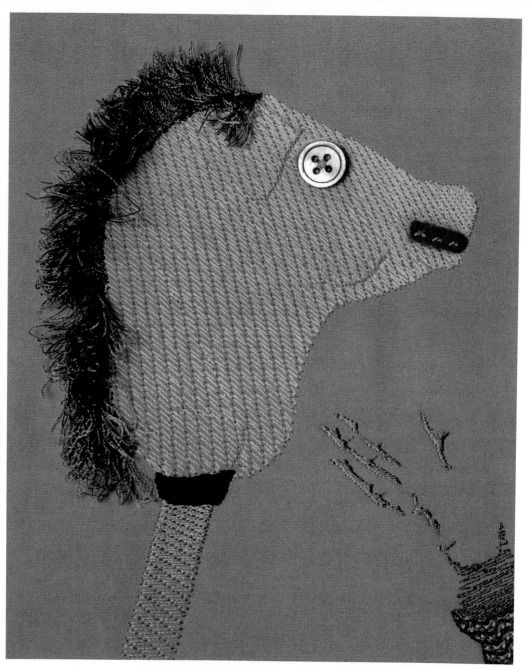

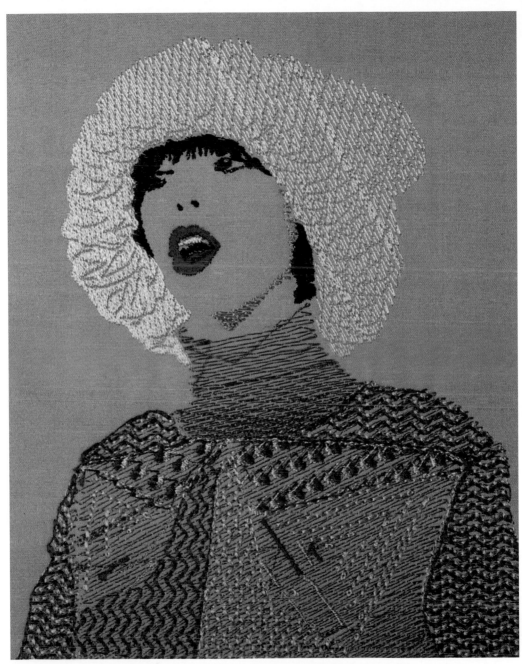

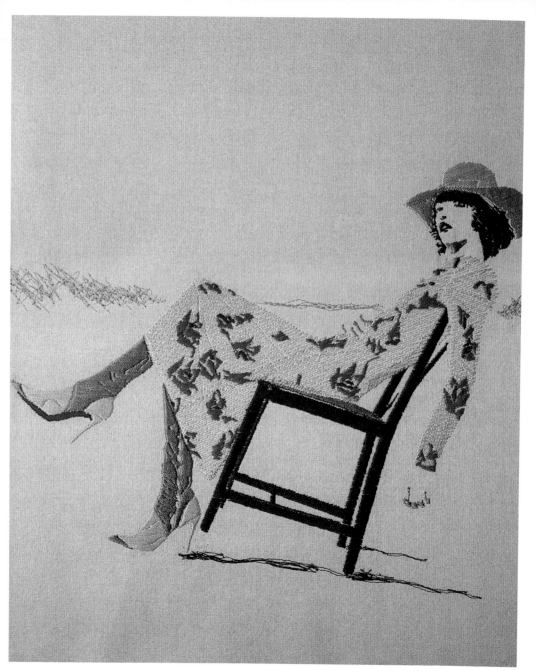

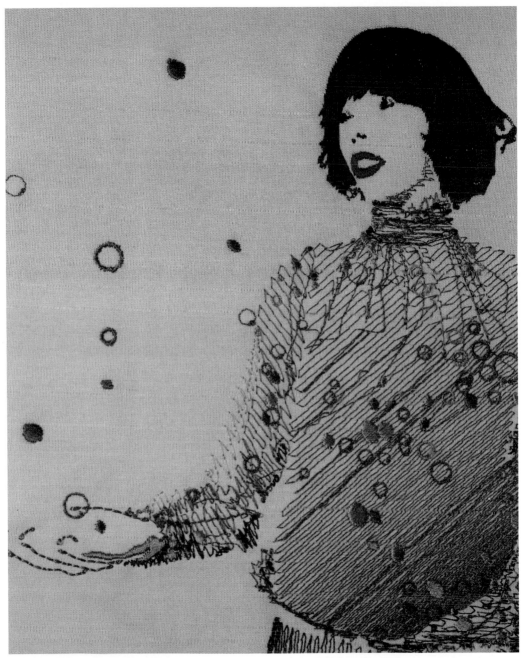

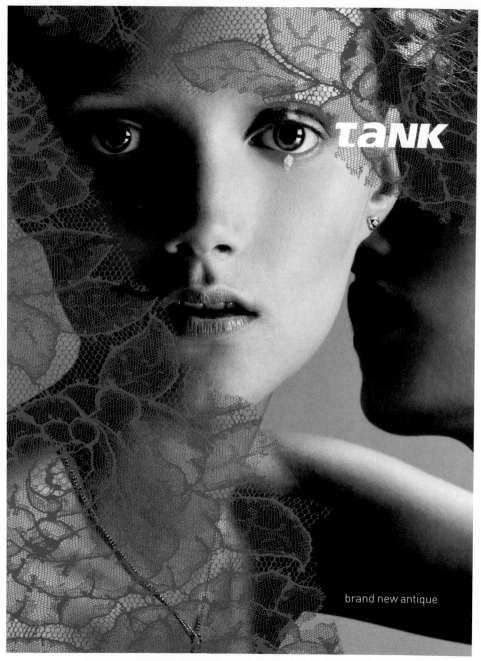

TANK

vol2 · issue 7 · £10

brand new antique

ELITISM FOR ALL

VOLUME 2 · ISSUE 7 · NOVEMBER 2001 · COVER PHOTOGRAPH BY ORION BEST

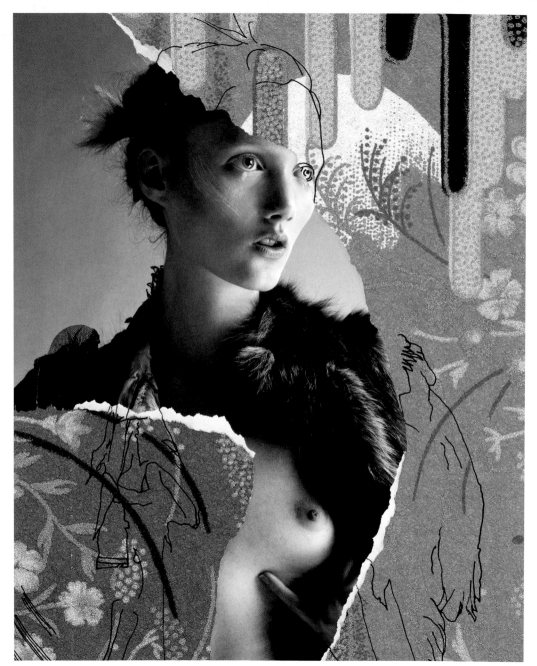

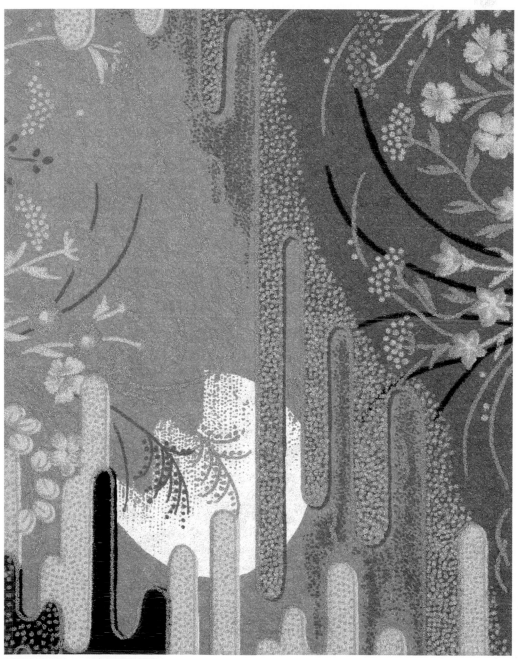

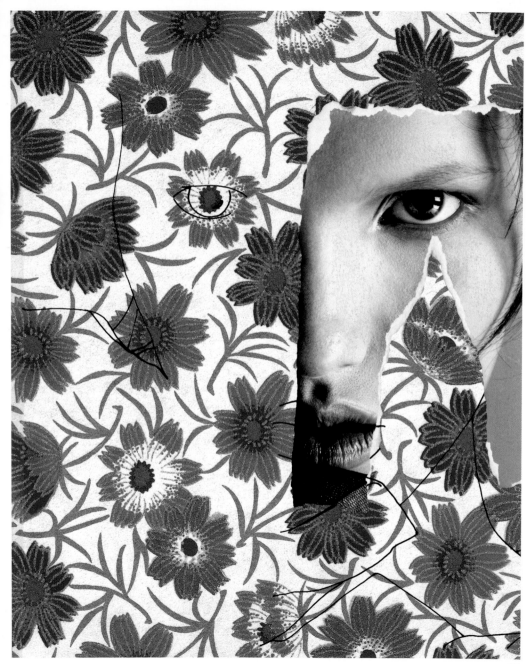

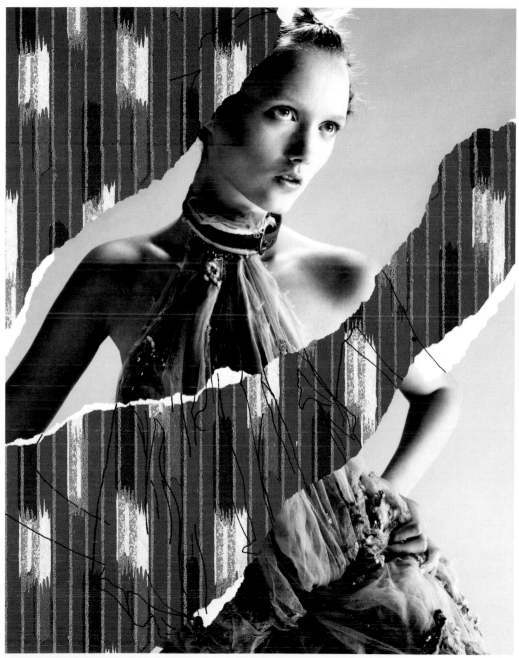

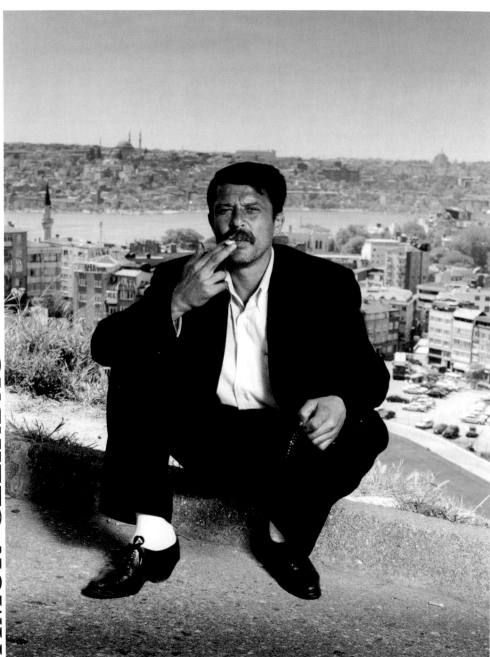

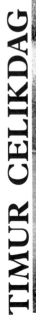

TIMUR CELIKDAG

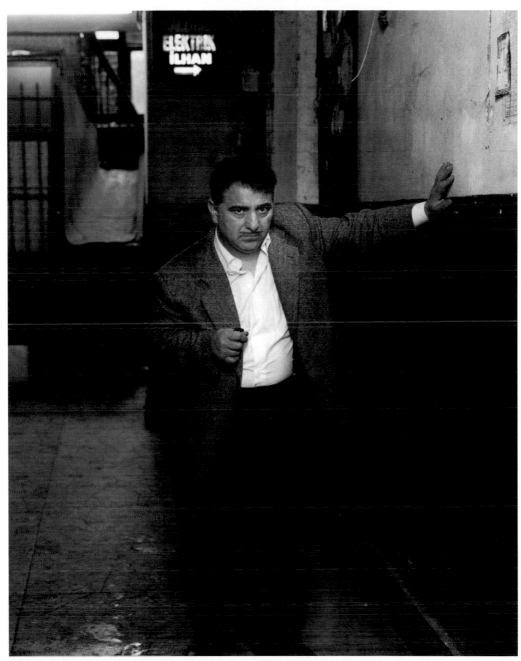

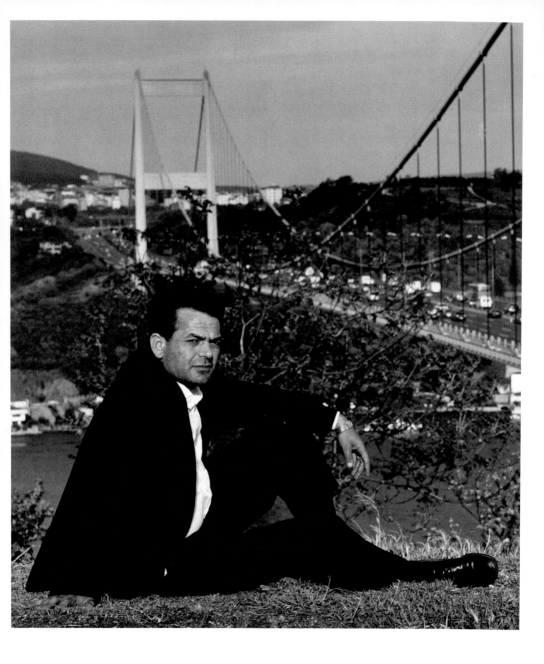

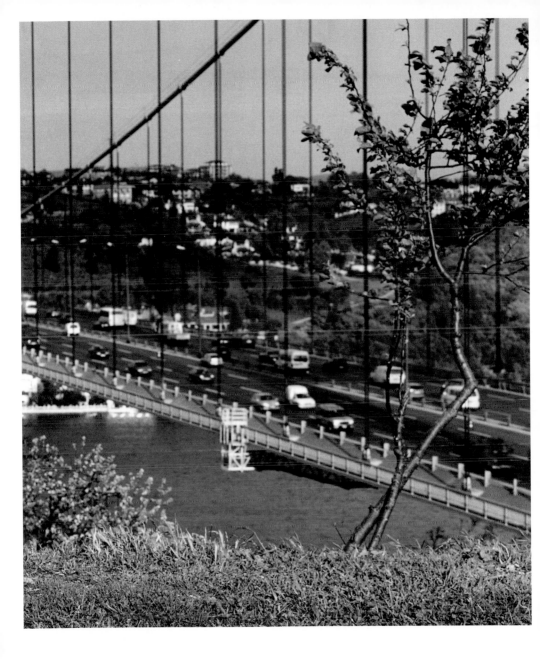

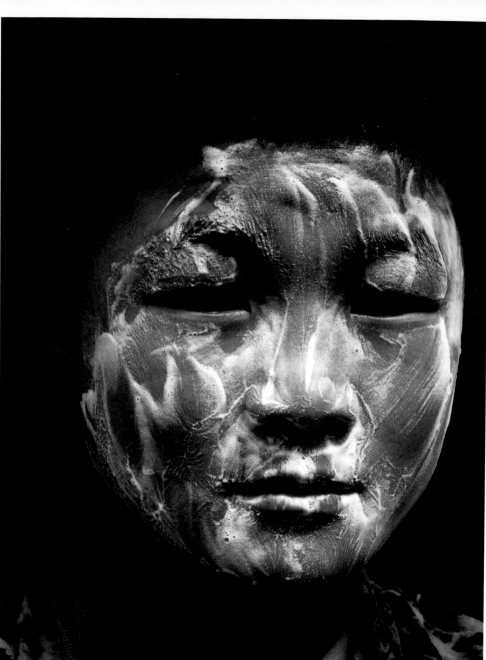

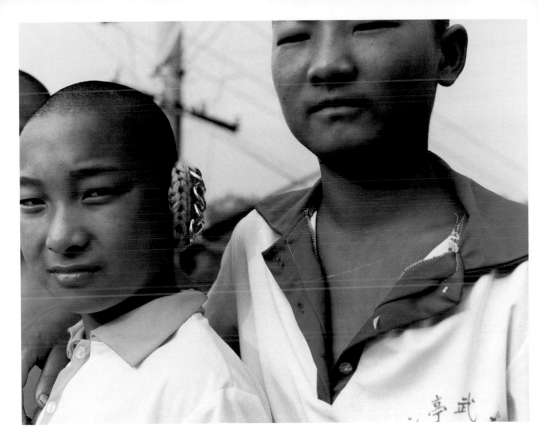

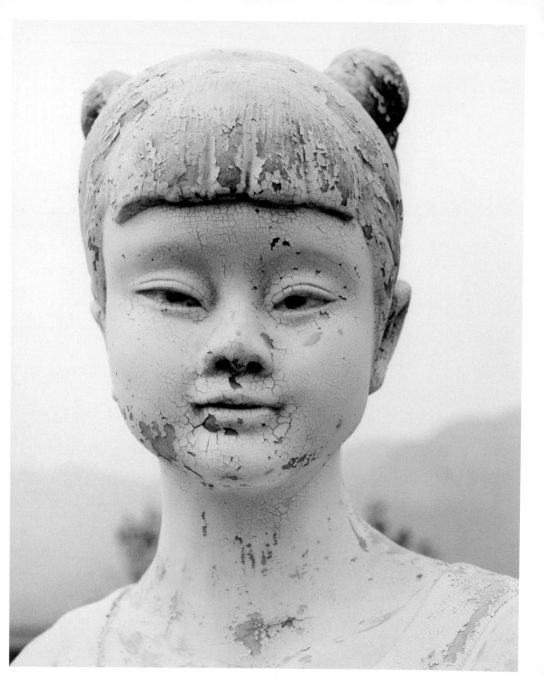

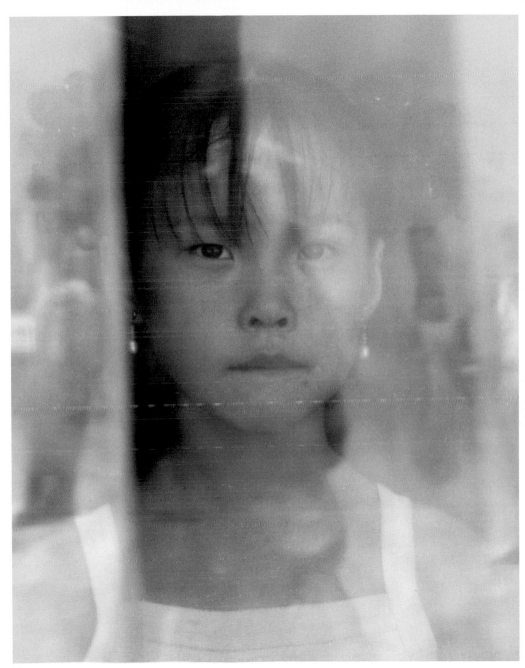

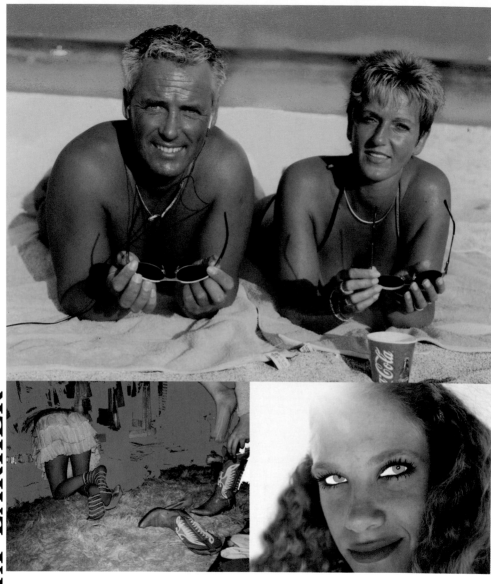

FELIX LARHER

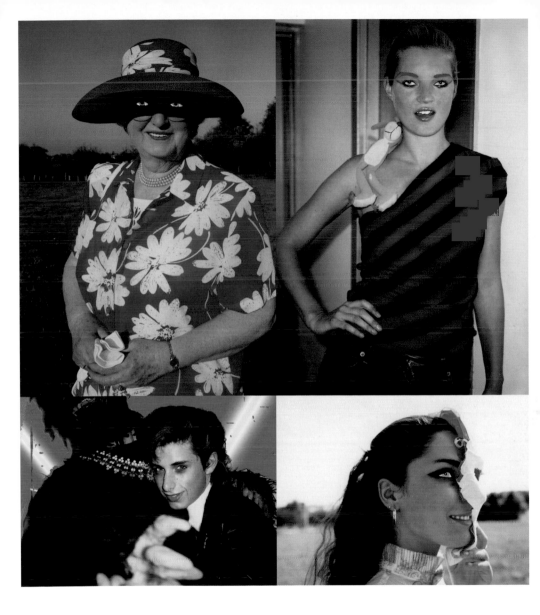

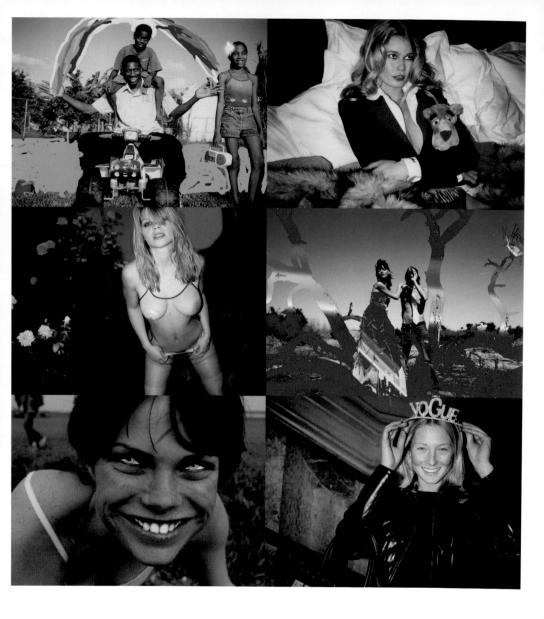

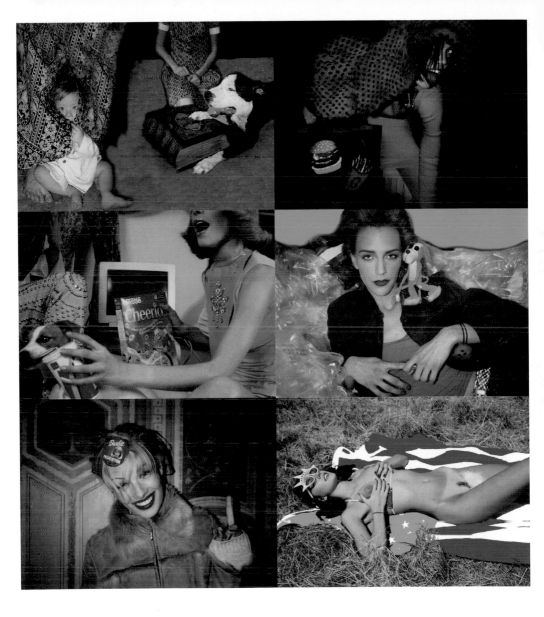

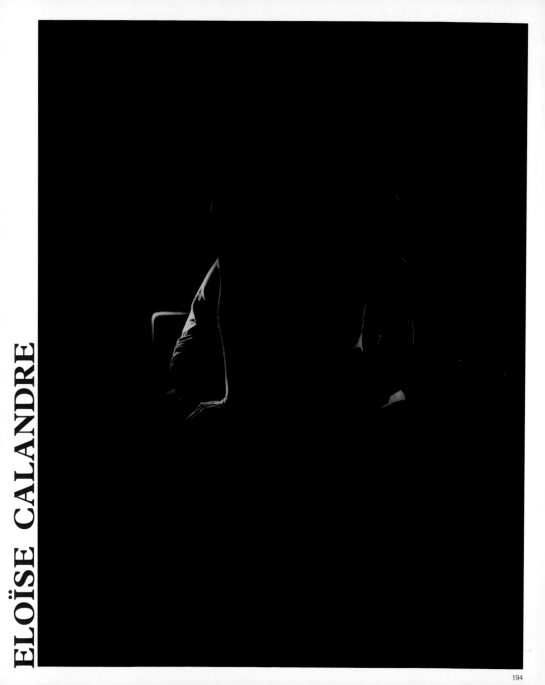

ELOÏSE CALANDRE

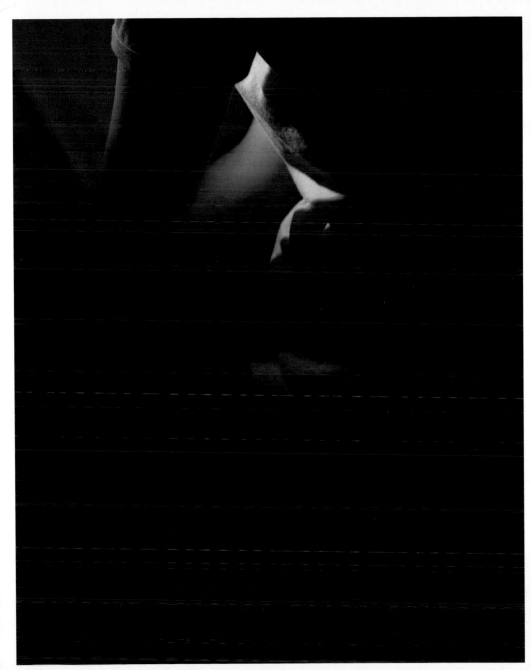

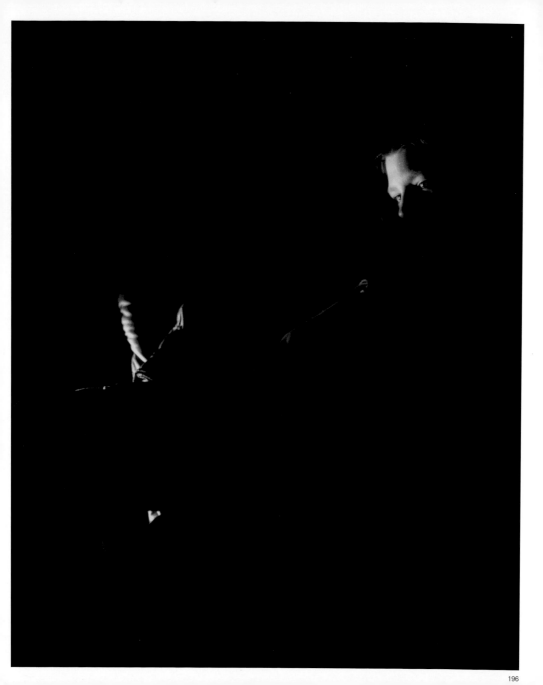

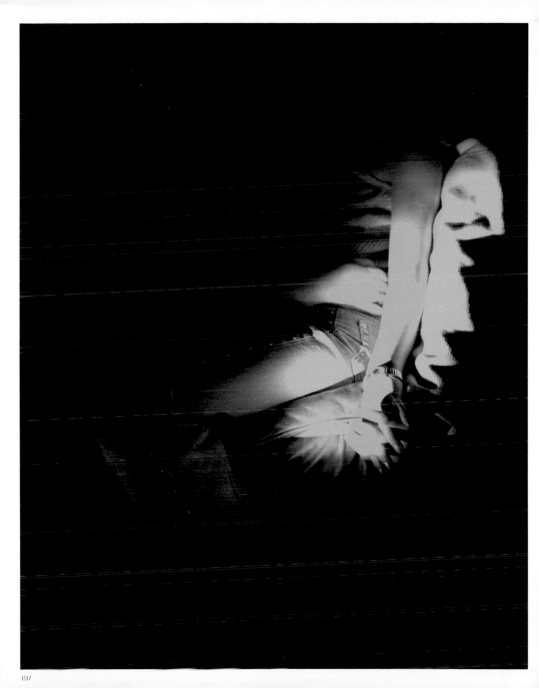

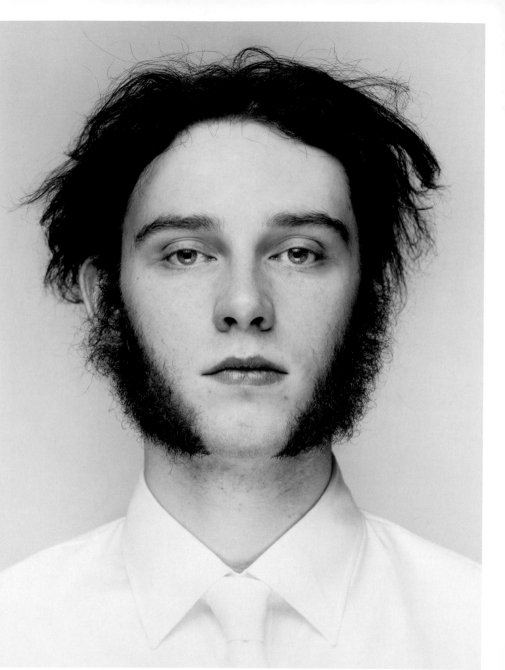

AXEL HOEDT

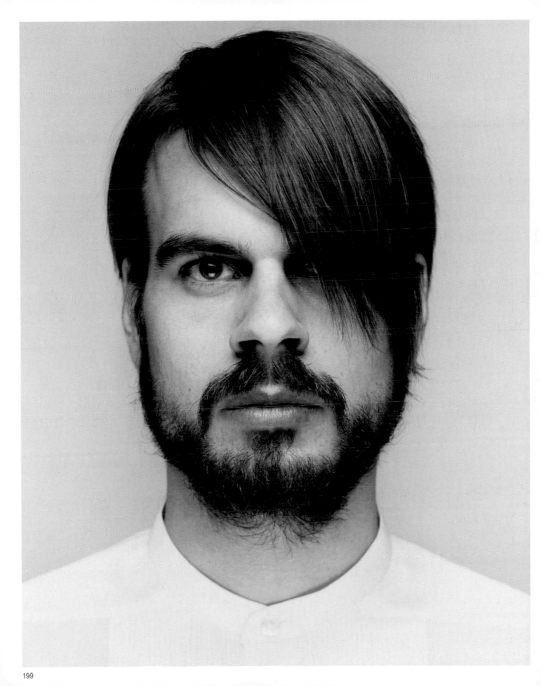

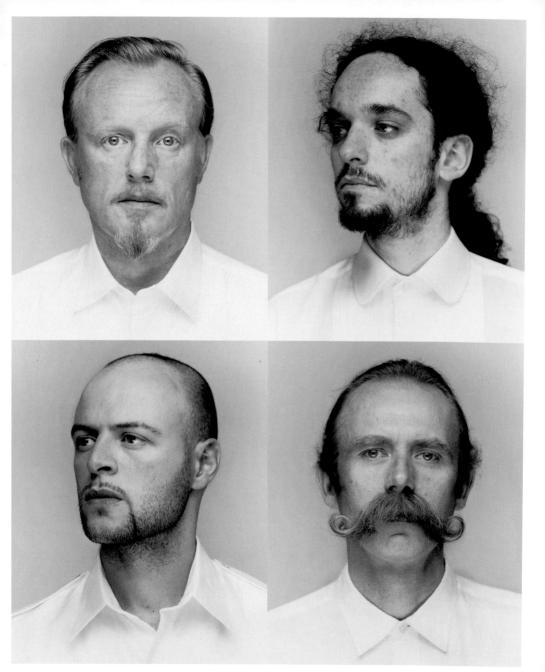

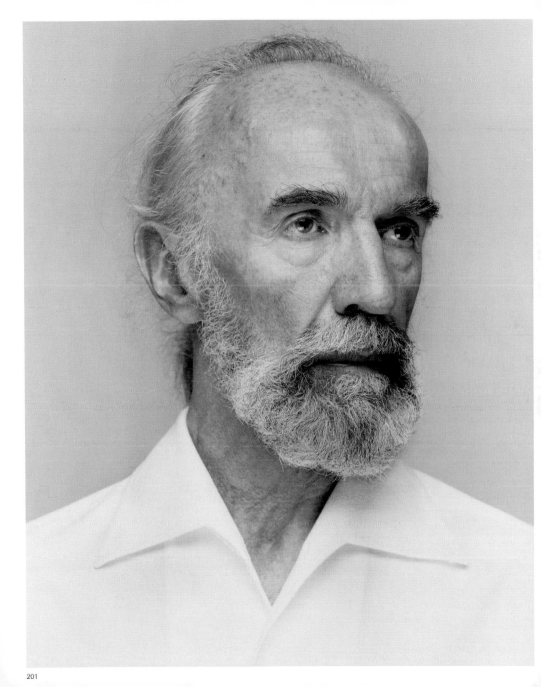

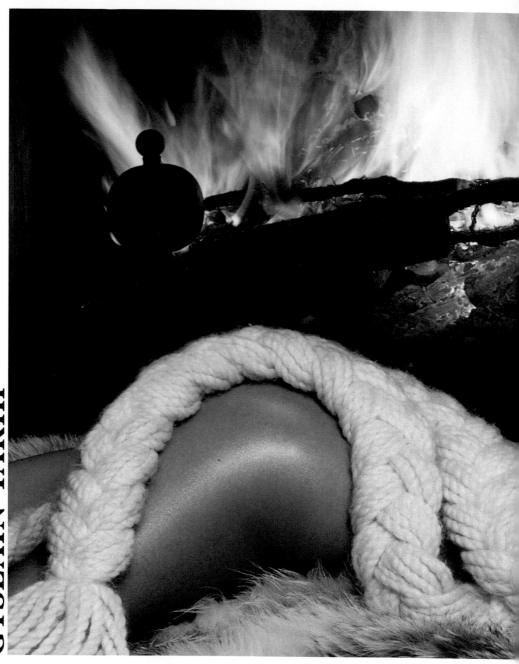

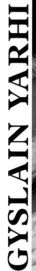

GYSLAIN YARHI

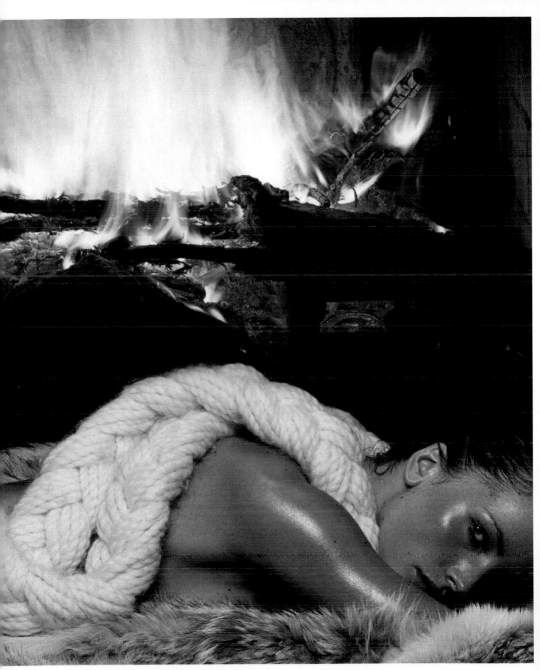

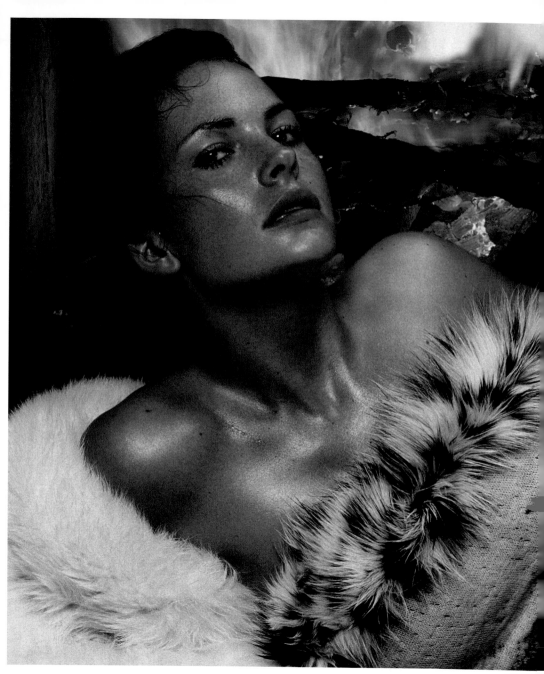

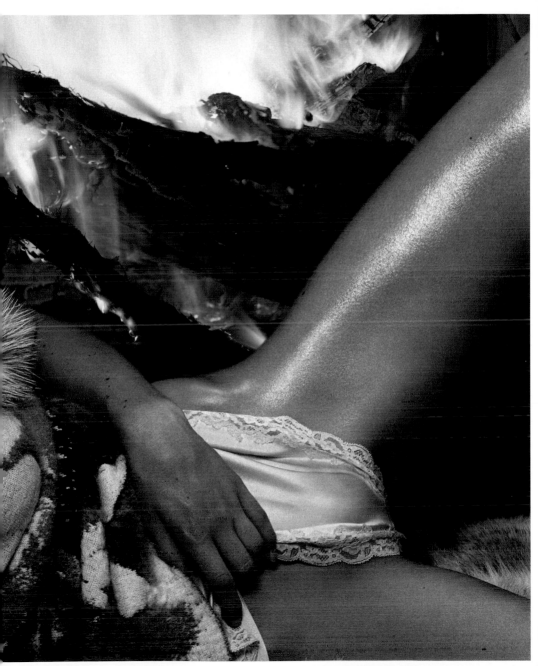

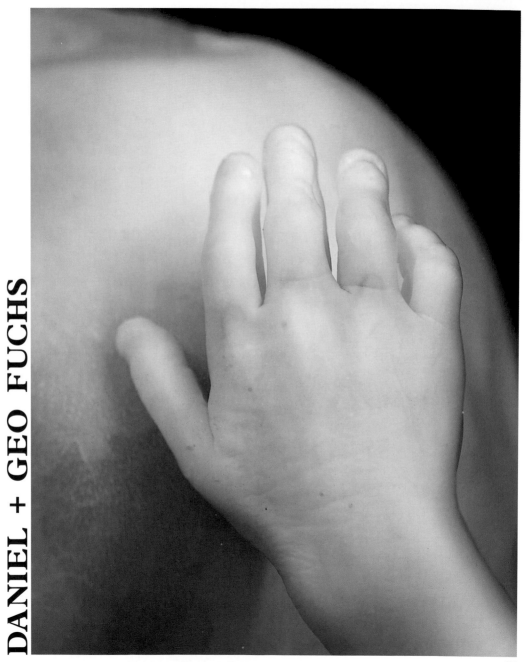

DANIEL + GEO FUCHS

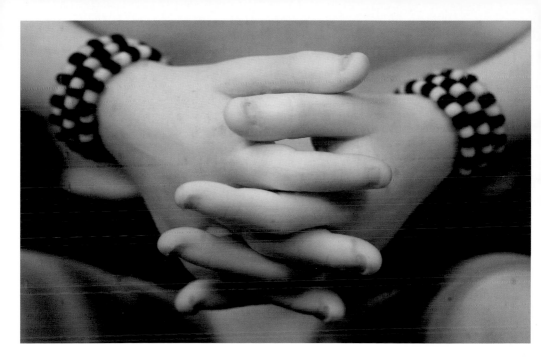

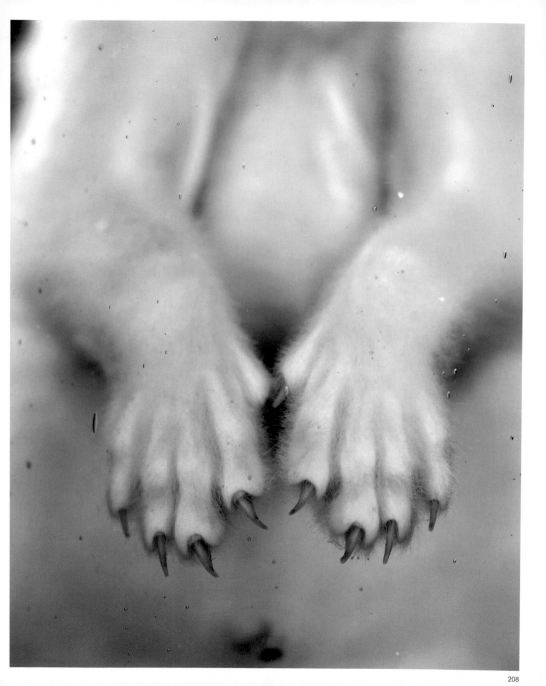

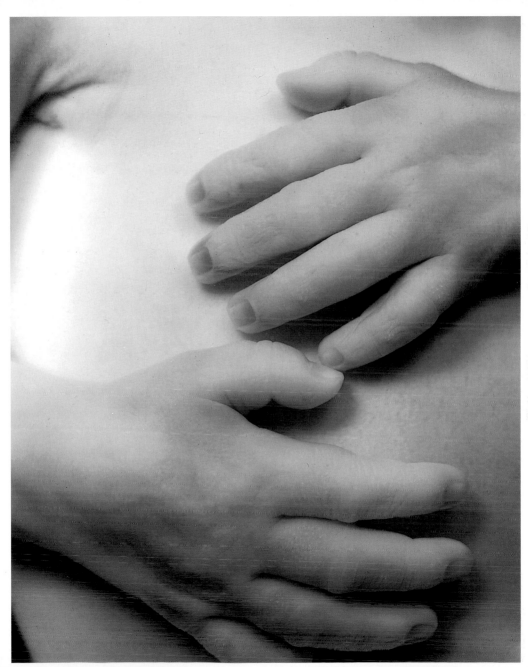

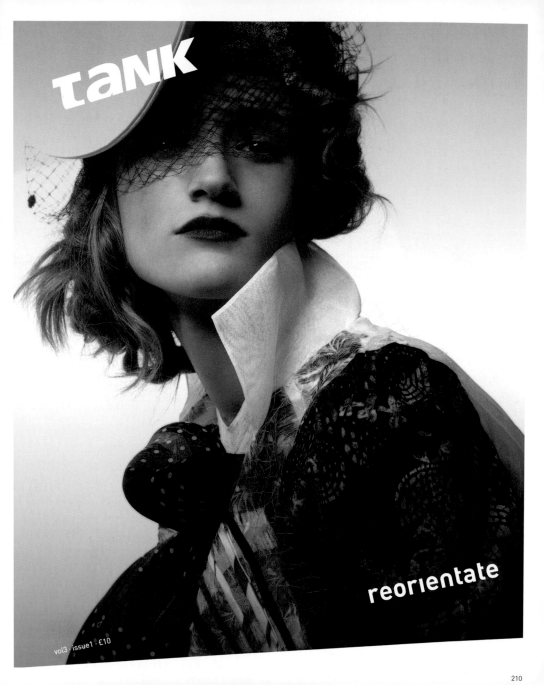

tank

reorientate

vol3 · issue1 · £10

DE STIJL · 100% PROOF

VOLUME 3 · ISSUE 1 · MARCH 2002 · COVER PHOTOGRAPH BY MASOUD

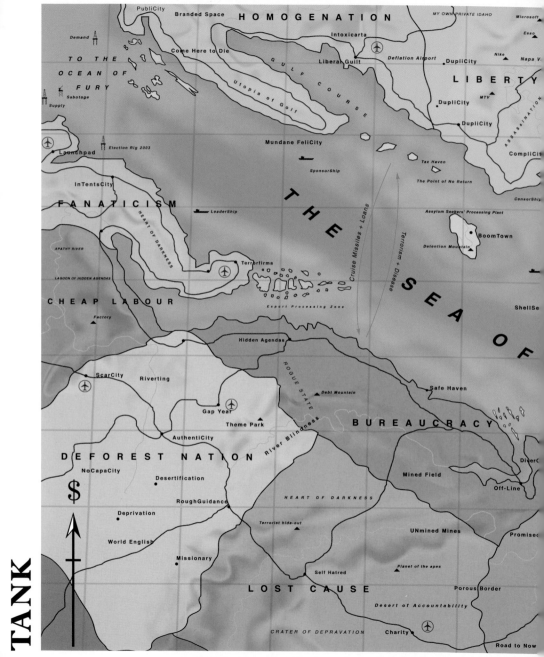

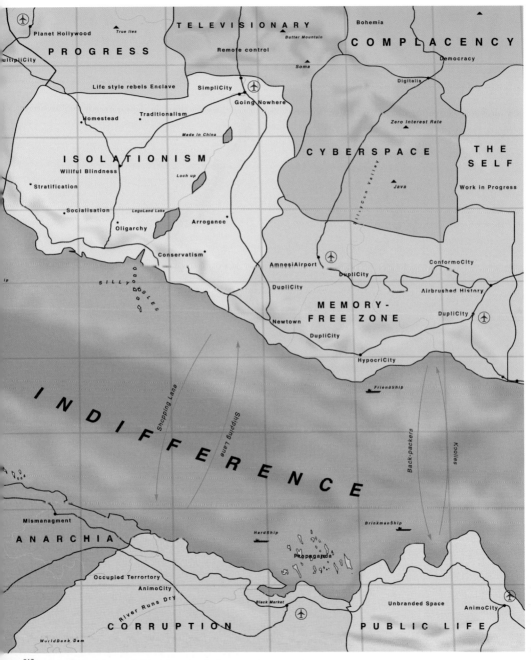

TELEVISIONARY

Bohemia

PROGRESS

COMPLACENCY

Planet Hollywood

True Iles

Butter Mountain

DupliCity

Remote control

Democracy

Soma

Digitalis

Life style rebels Enclave

SimpliCity

Going Nowhere

Homestead

Traditionalism

Zero Interest Rate

Made in China

ISOLATIONISM

CYBERSPACE

THE SELF

Willful Blindness

Loch up

Java

Work in Progress

Stratification

Socialisation

LegoLand Lake

Oligarchy

Arrogance

Conservatism

AmnesiAirport

ConformoCity

DupliCity

Airbrushed History

ip

SILLY DOSLES

DupliCity

MEMORY-FREE ZONE

DupliCity

Newtown

DupliCity

HypocriCity

Shopping Lane

Shopping Lane

Back-packers

Koolies

FriendShip

INDIFFERENCE

Mismanagment

BrinkmanShip

ANARCHIA

HardShip

Occupied Terrortory

Propaganda

AnimoCity

River Runs Dry

Black Market

Unbranded Space

AnimoCity

CORRUPTION

PUBLIC LIFE

WorldBank Dam

213

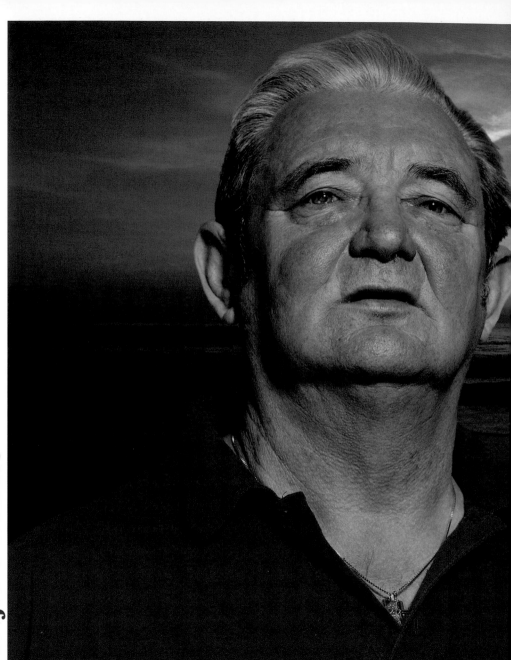

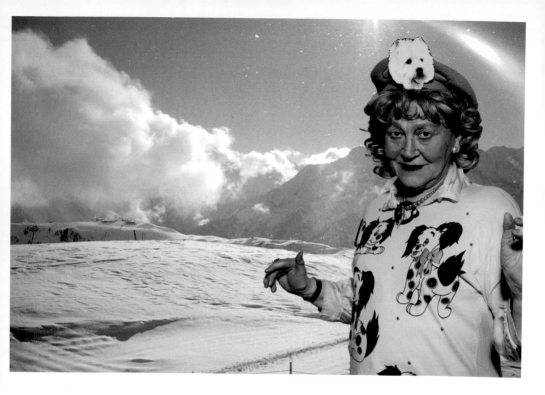

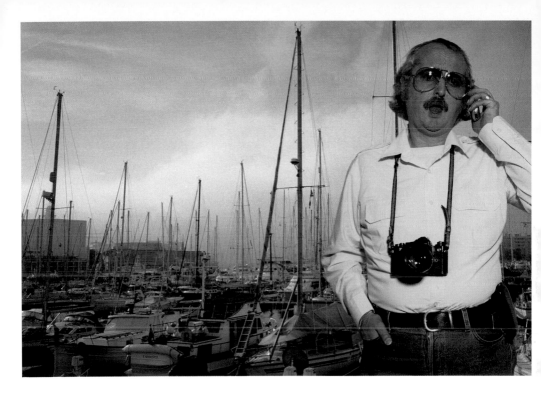

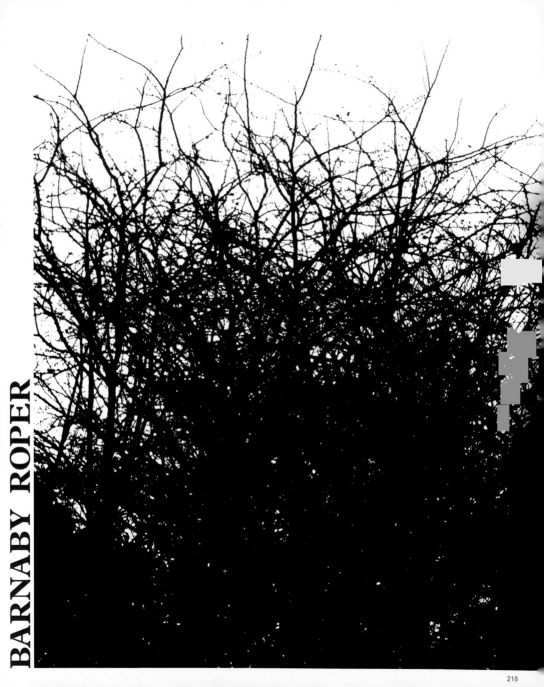

BARNABY ROPER

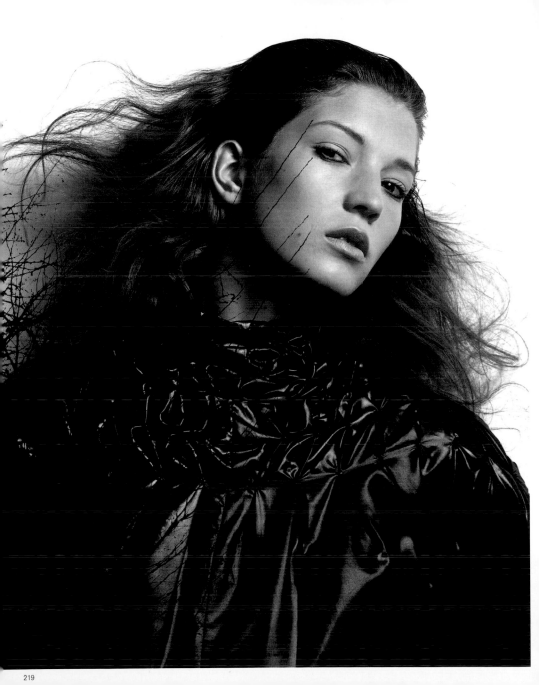

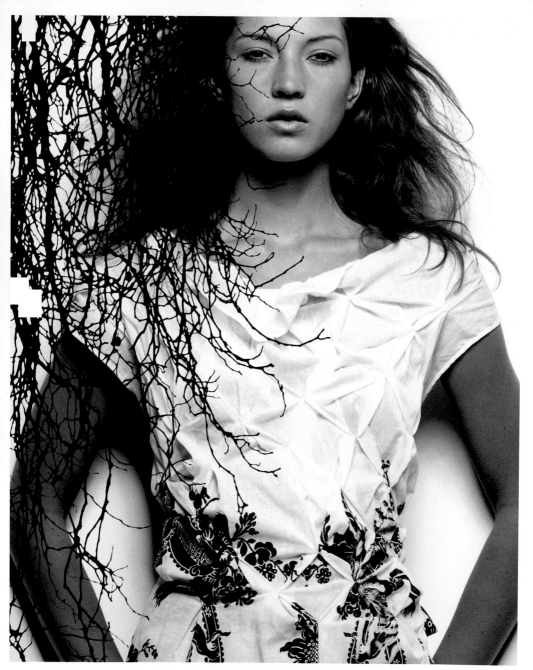

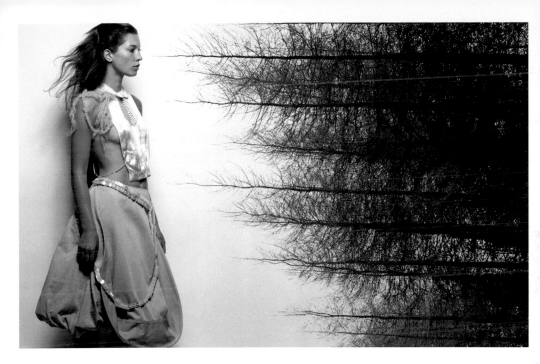

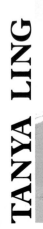

TANYA LING

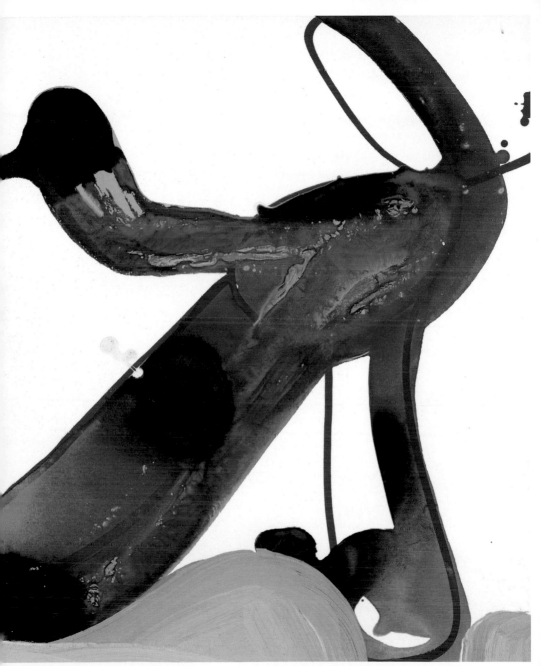

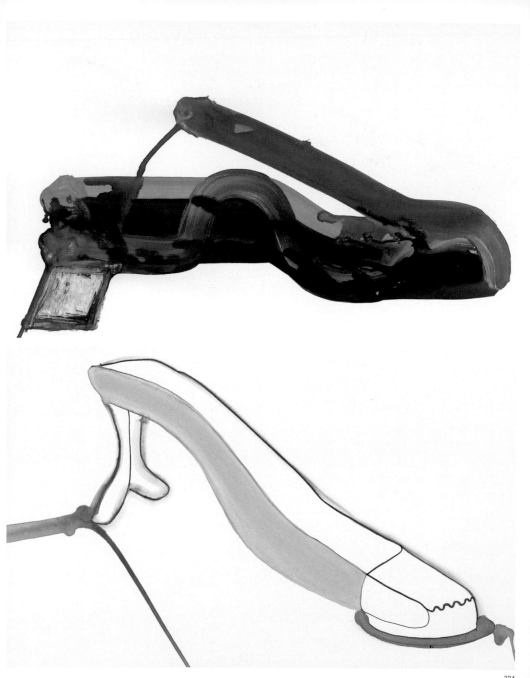

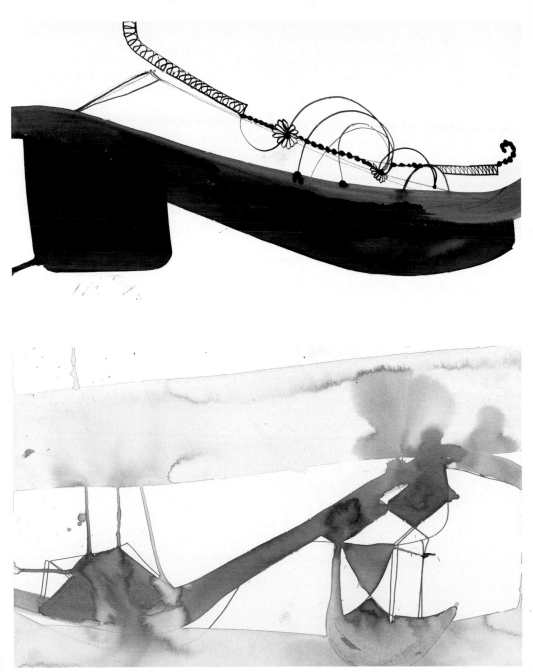

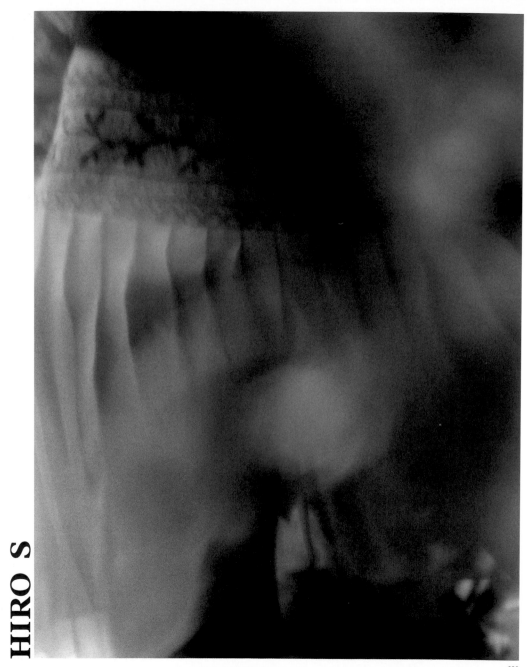

HIRO S

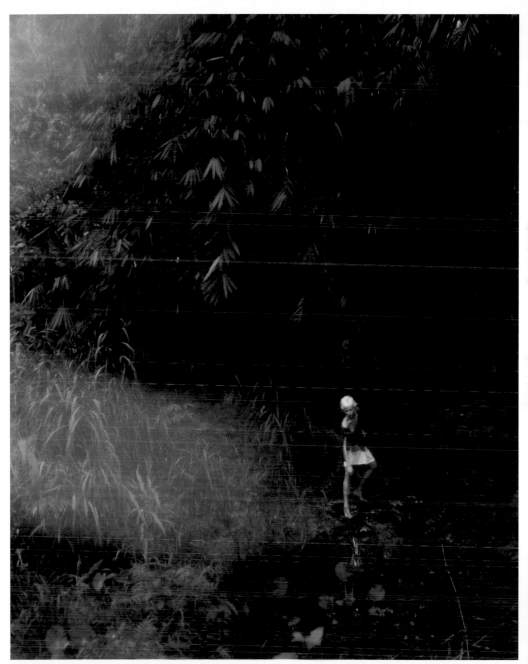

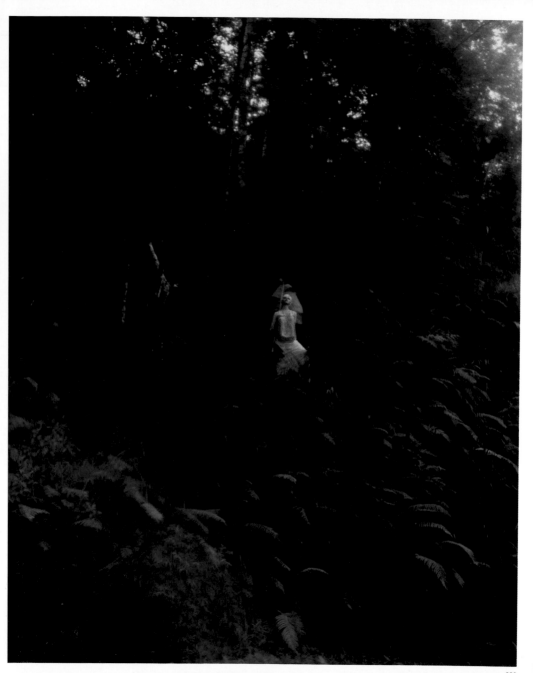

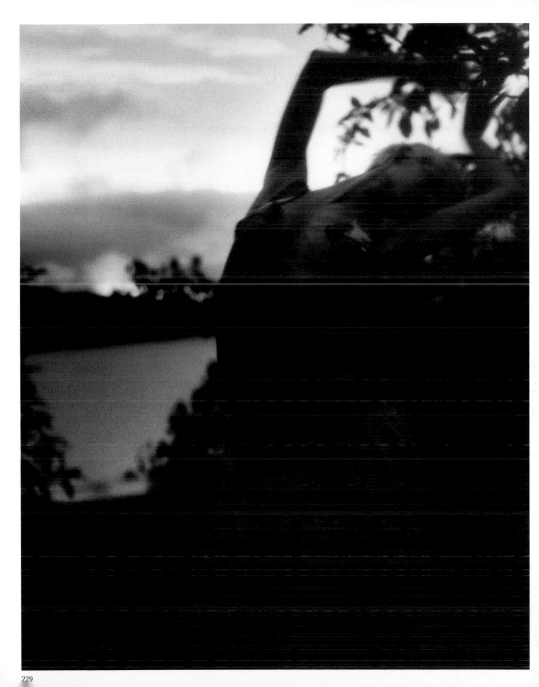

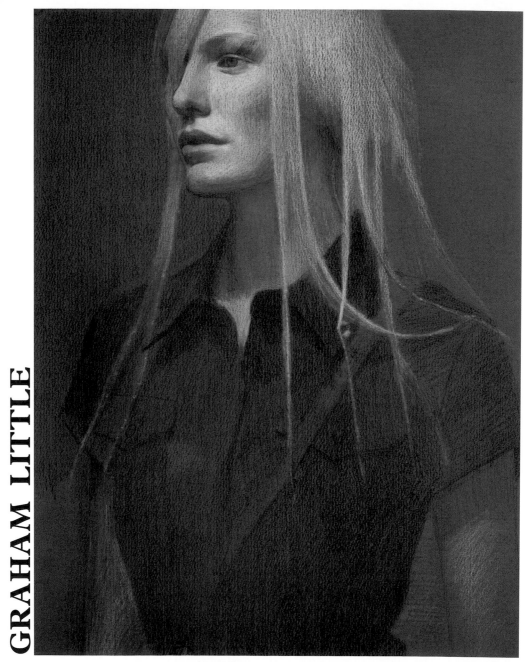

GRAHAM LITTLE

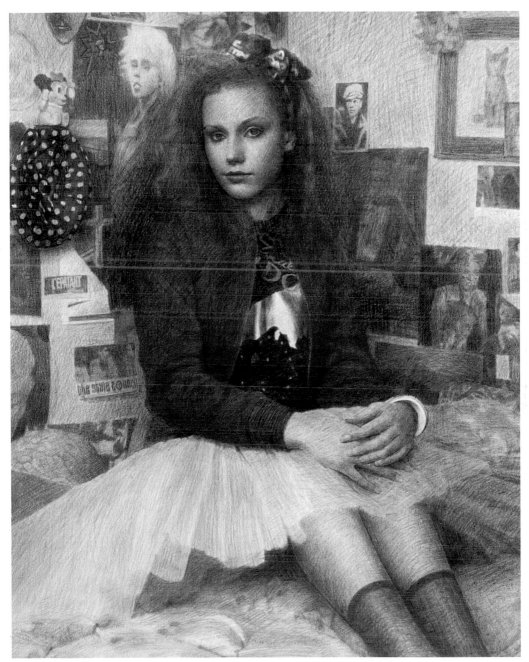

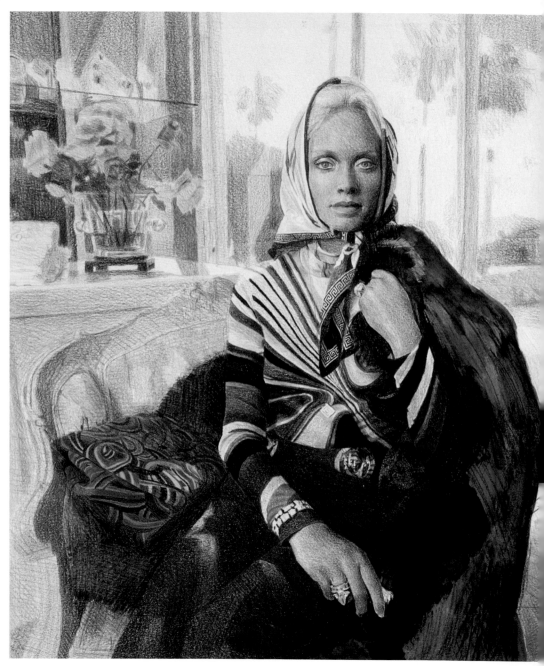

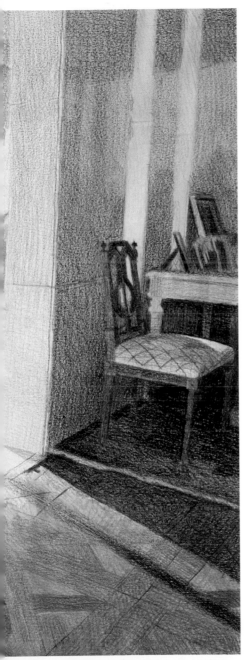

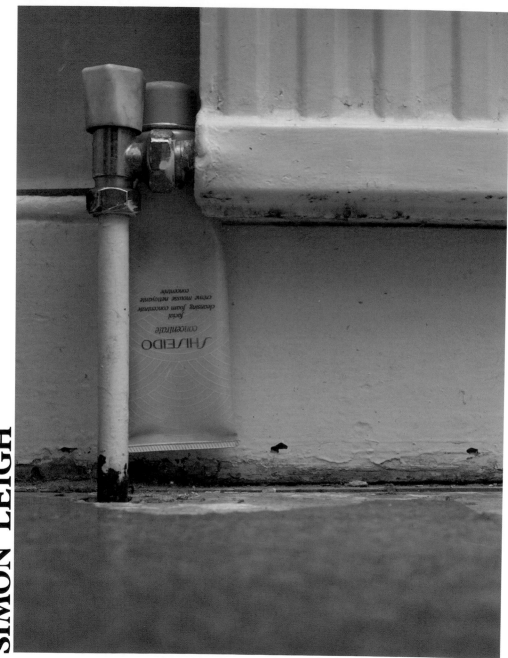

SIMON LEIGH

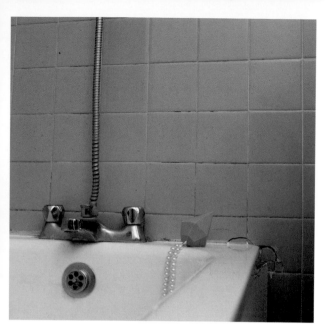

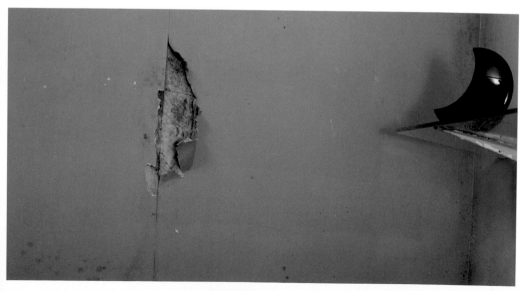

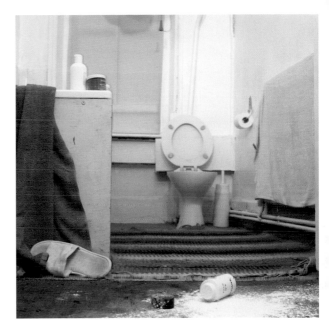

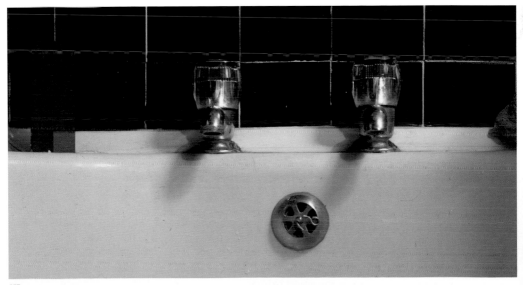

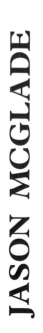

JASON MCGLADE

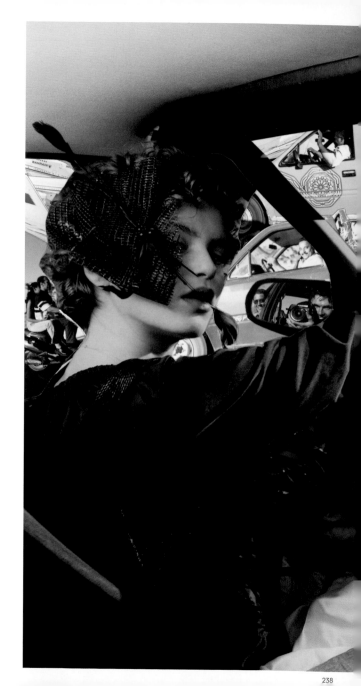

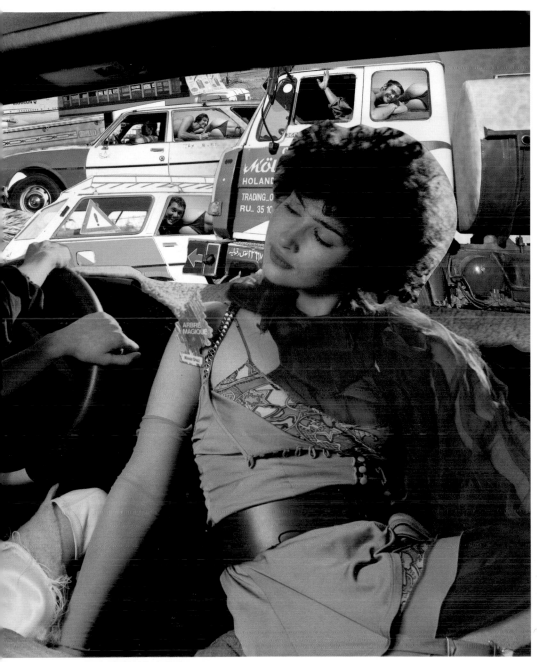

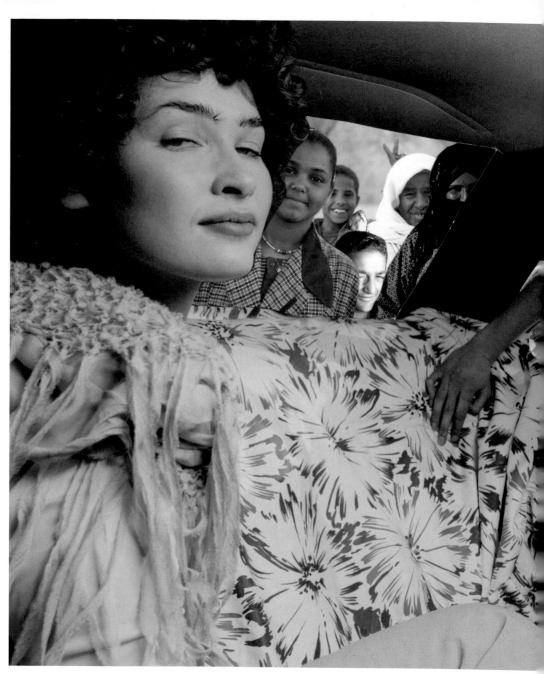

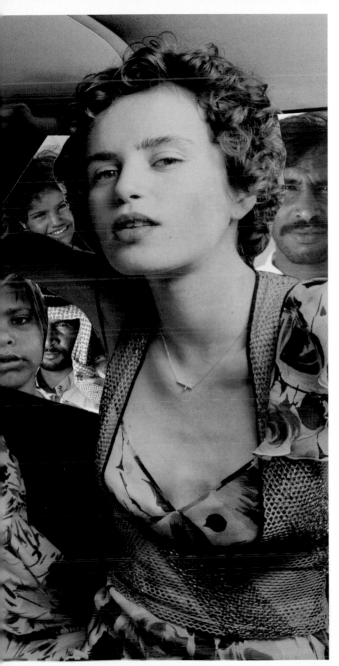

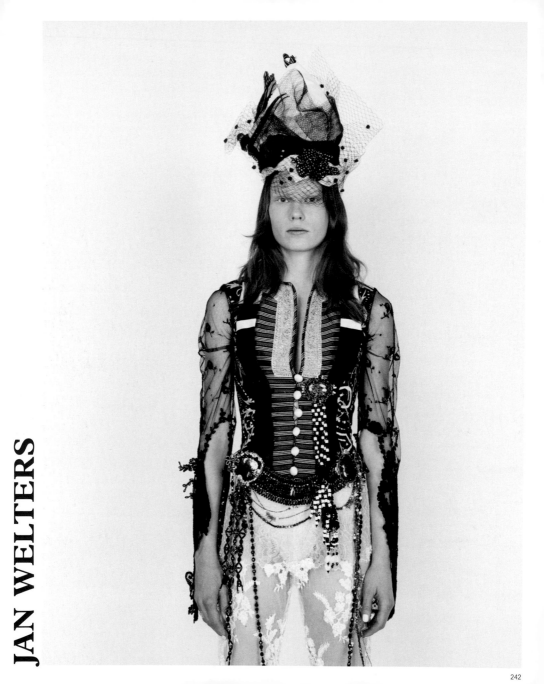

JAN WELTERS

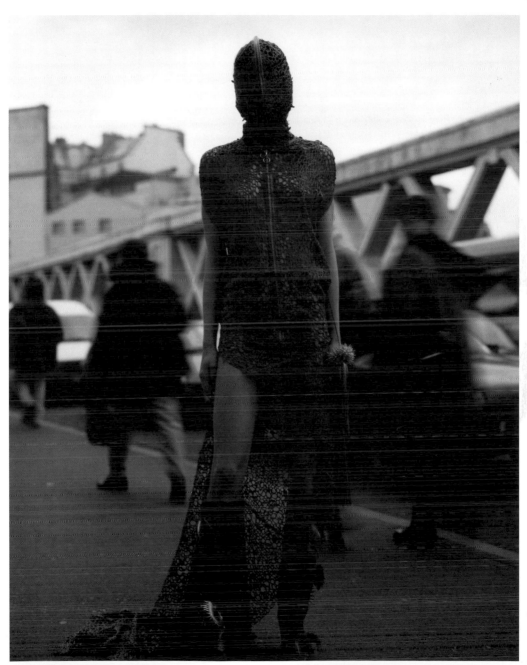

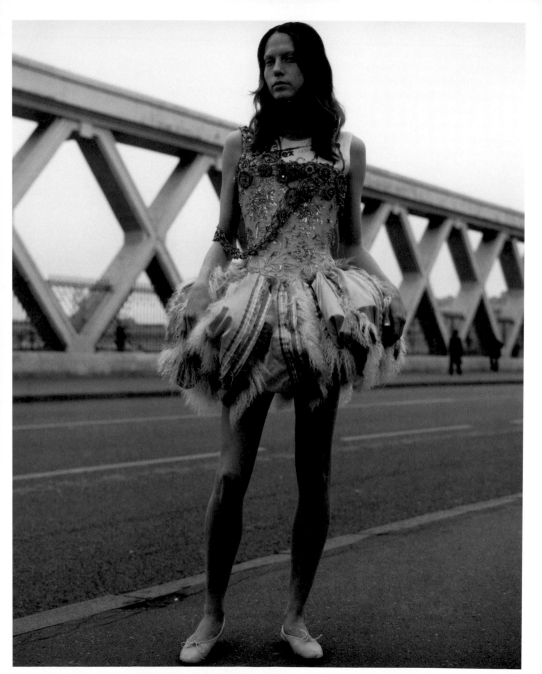

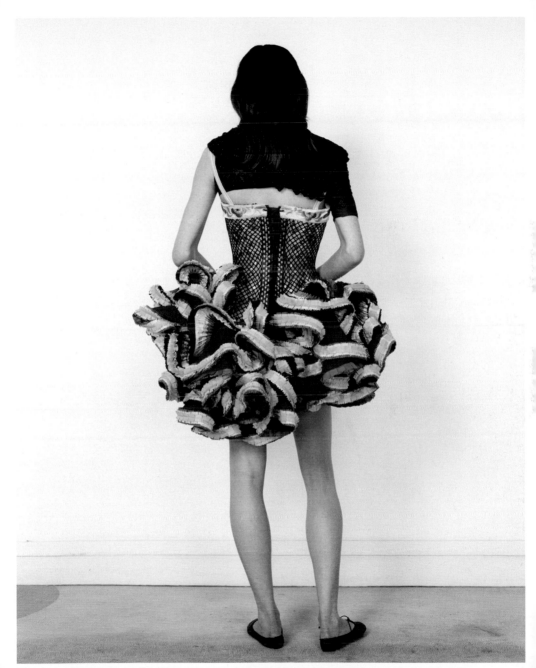

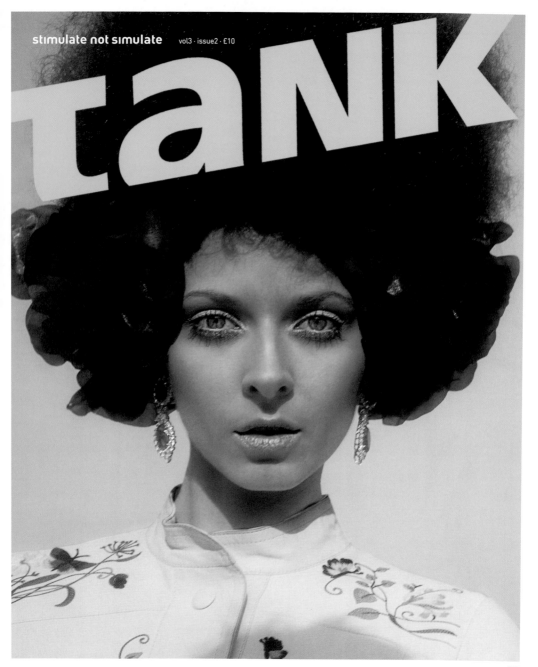

TANK

ACTUAL REALITY

VOLUME 3 · ISSUE 2 · JUNE 2002 · COVER PHOTOGRAPH BY LOUIS DECAMPS

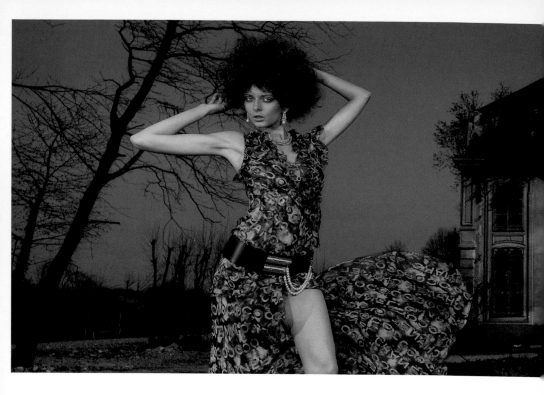

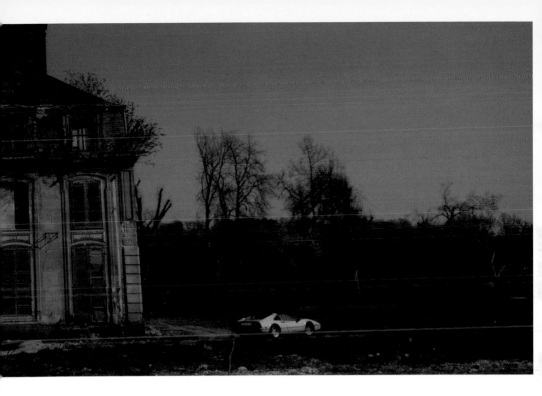

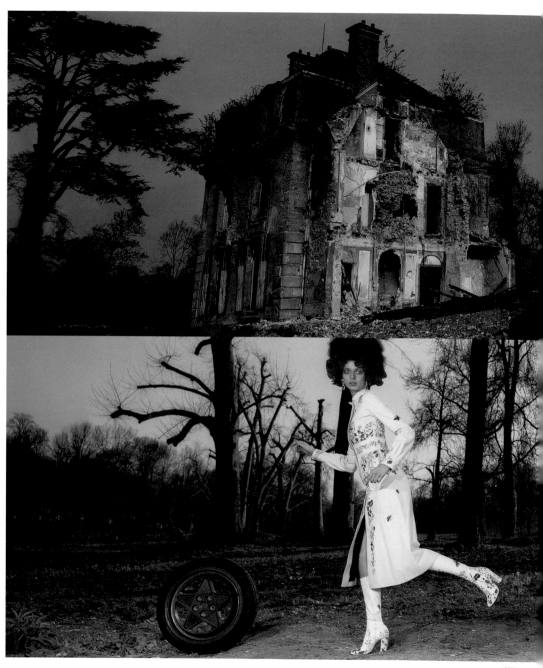

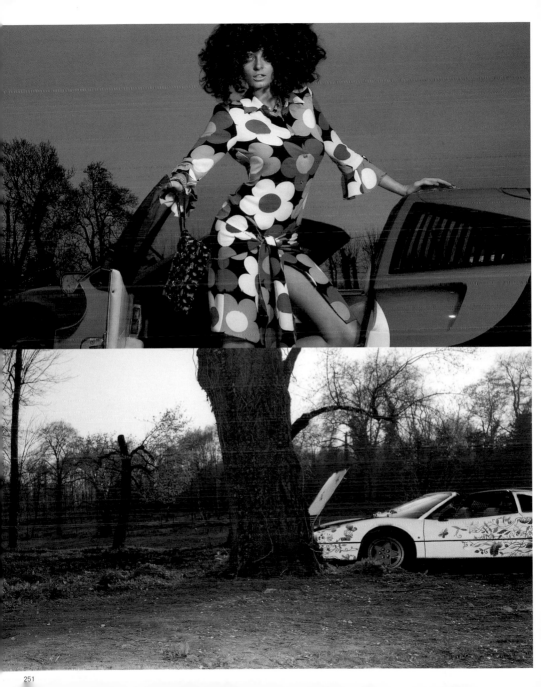

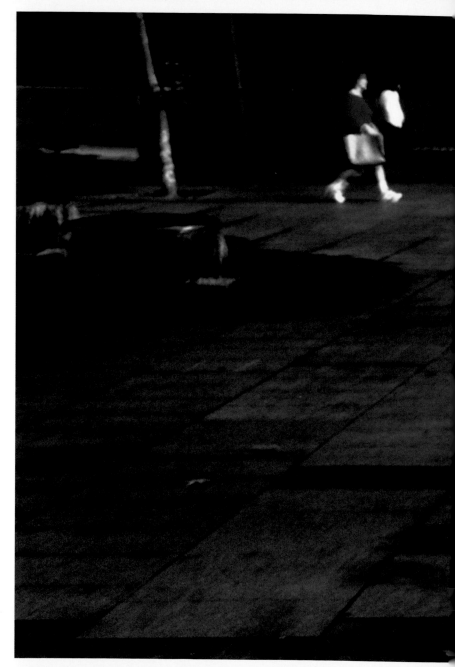

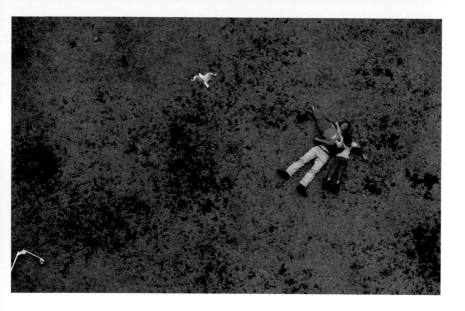

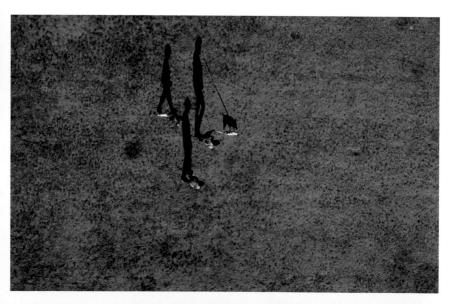

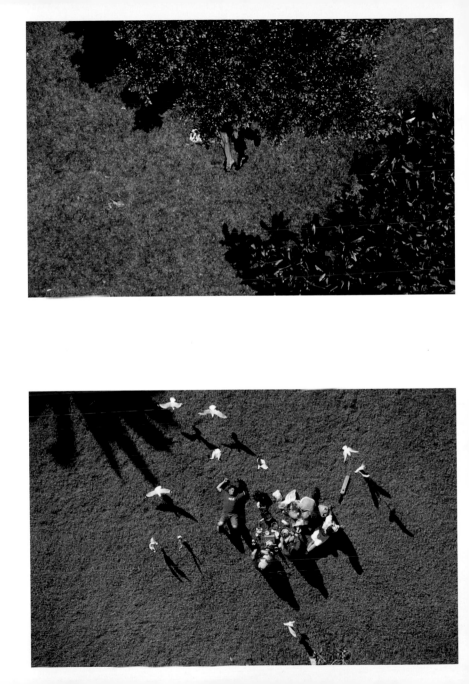

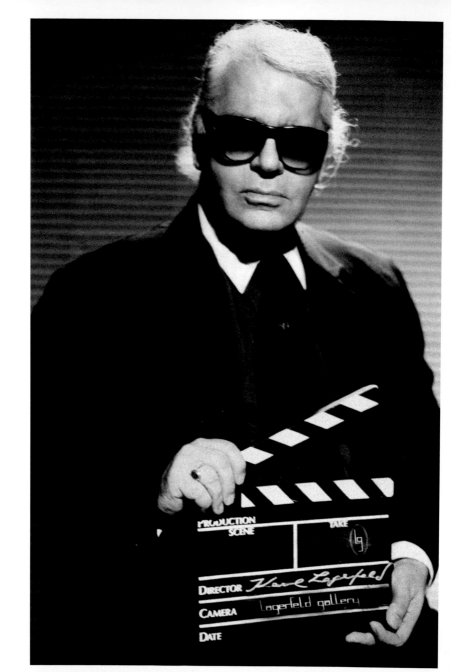

ALI MAHDAVI

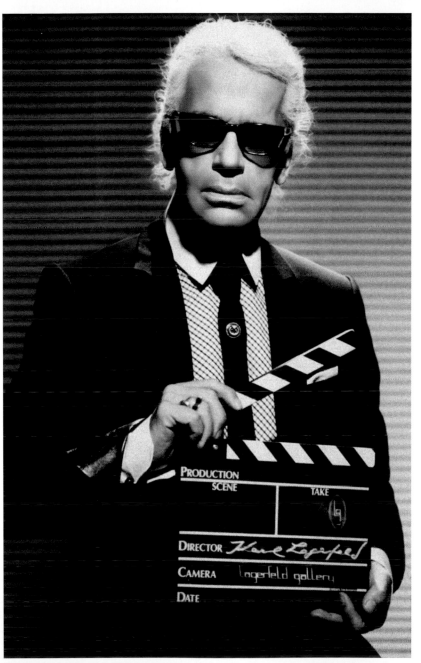

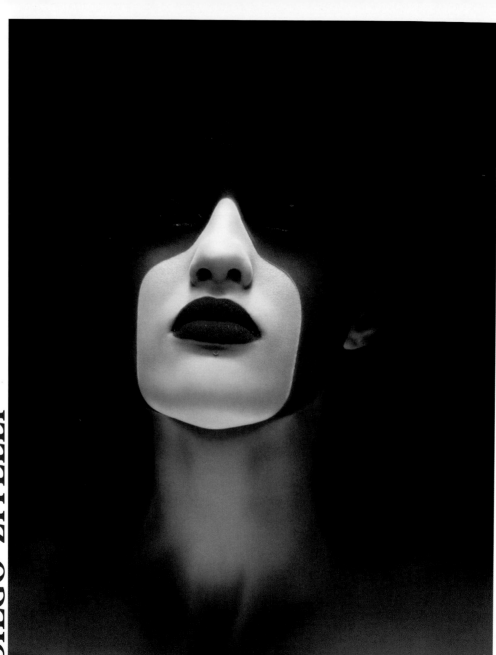

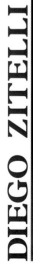
DIEGO ZITELLI

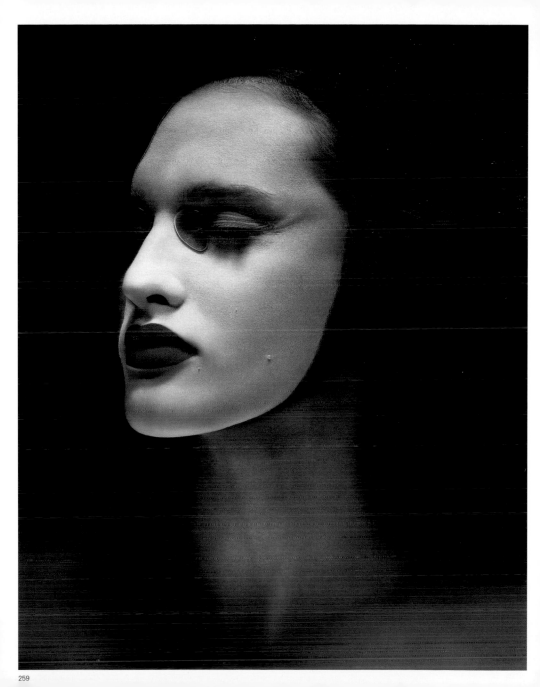

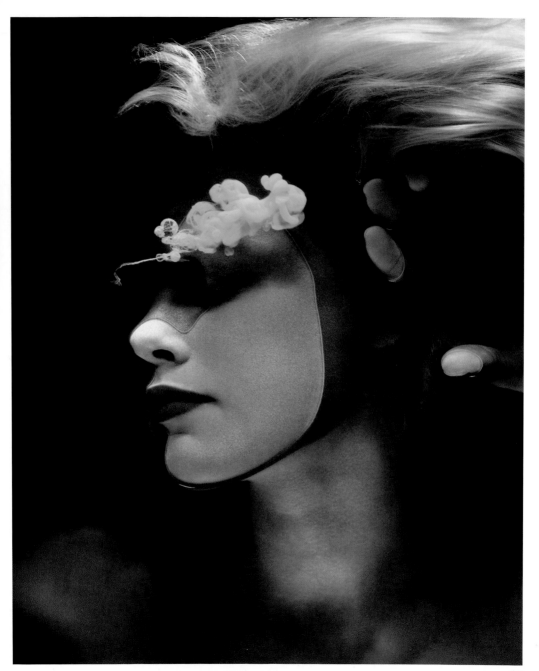

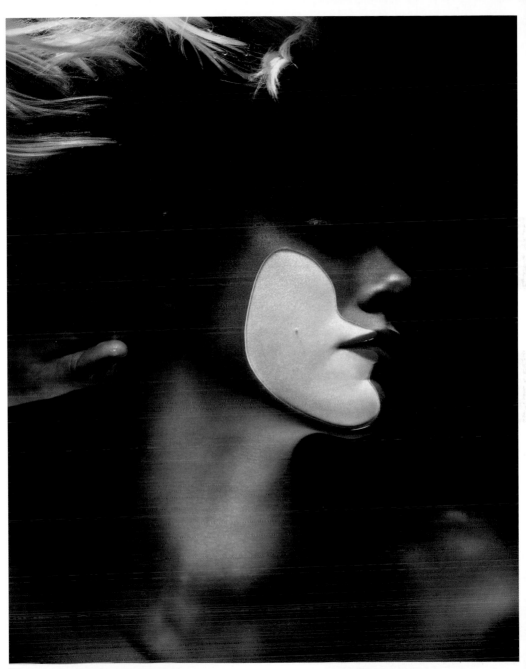

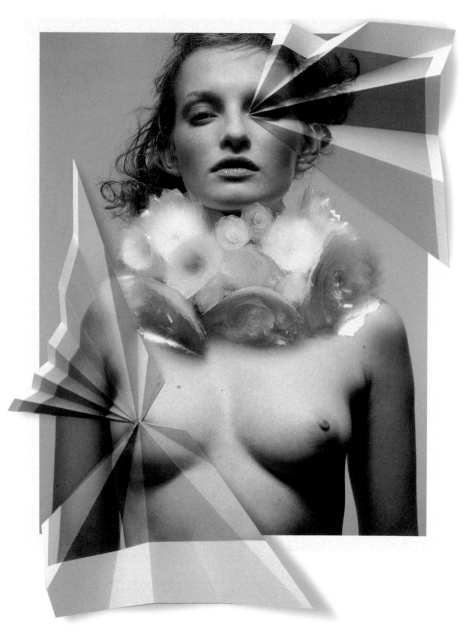

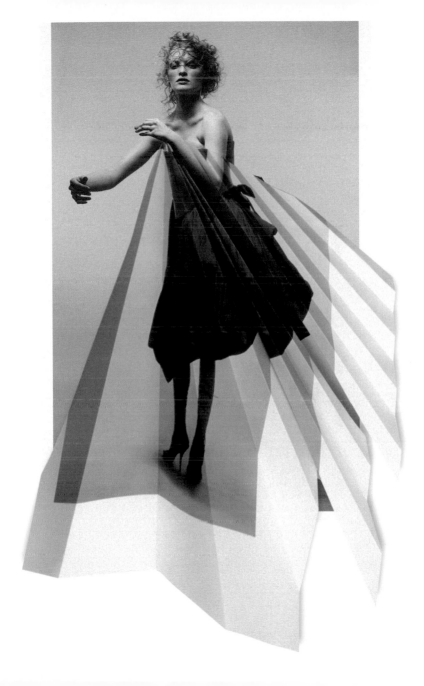

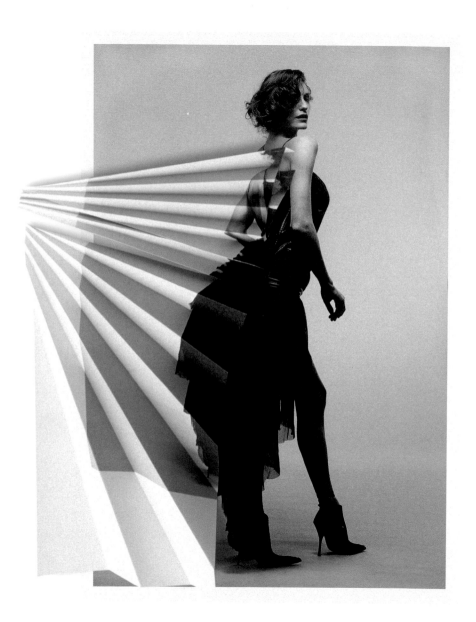

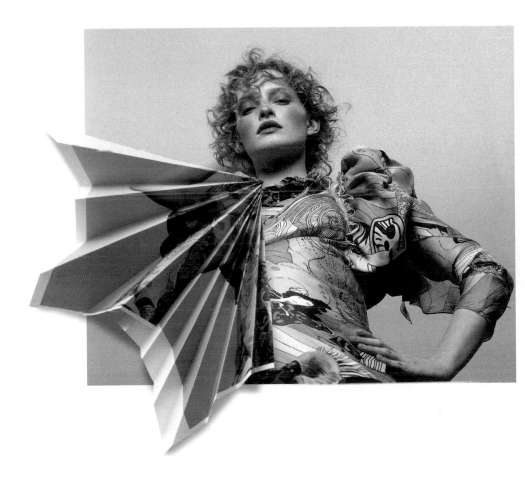

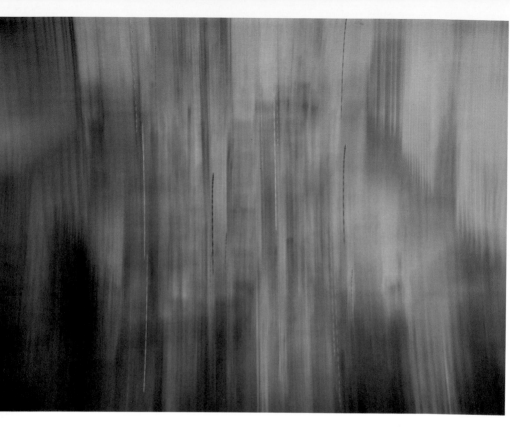

CATHERINE YASS

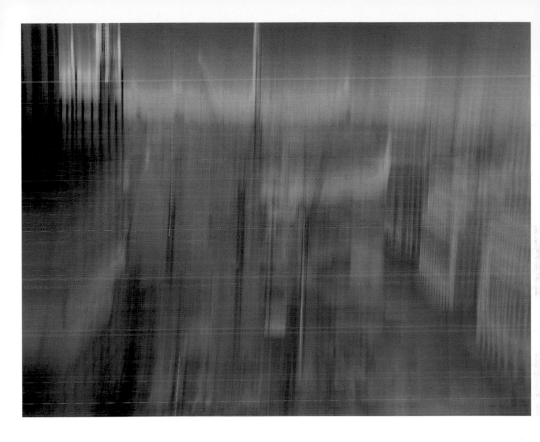

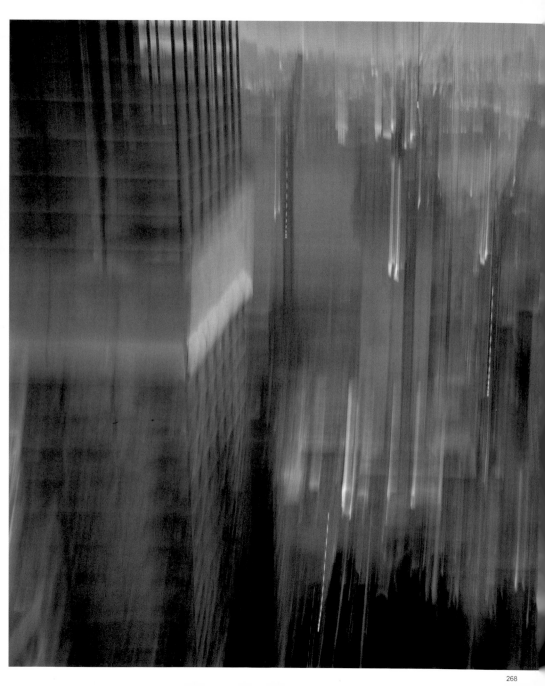

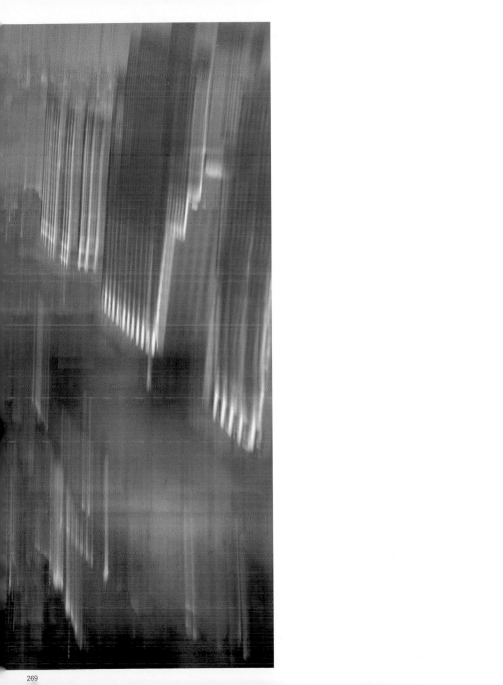

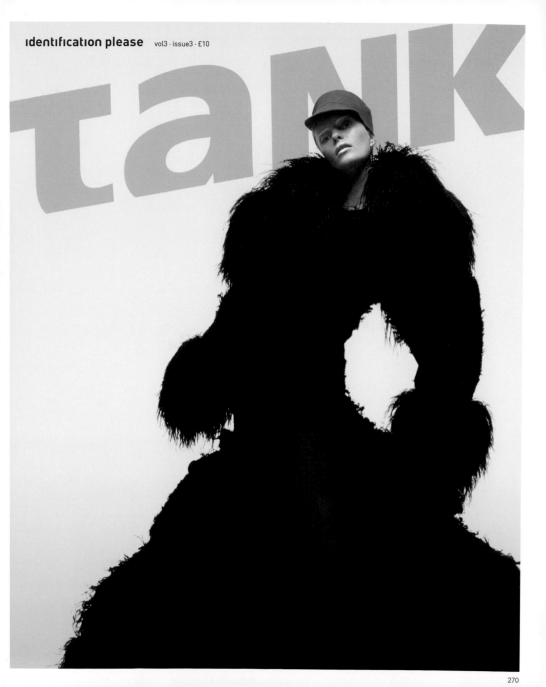

identification please   vol3 · issue3 · £10

TANK

POST-SCRIPT

VOLUME 3 · ISSUE 3 · SEPTEMBER 2002 · COVER PHOTOGRAPH BY MASOUD

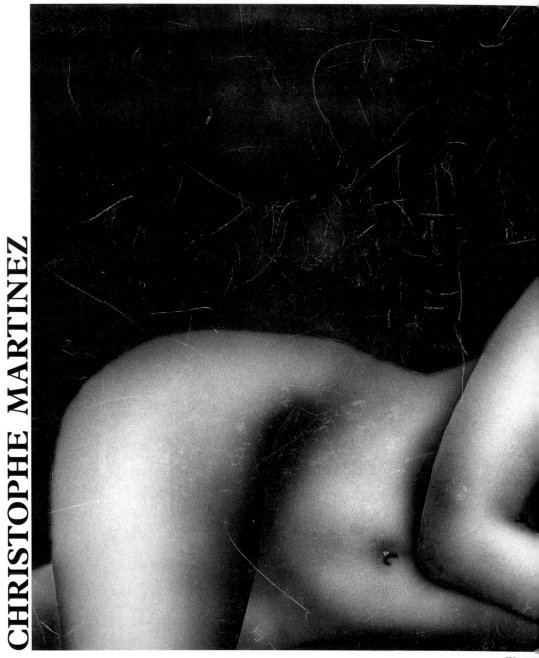

CHRISTOPHE MARTINEZ

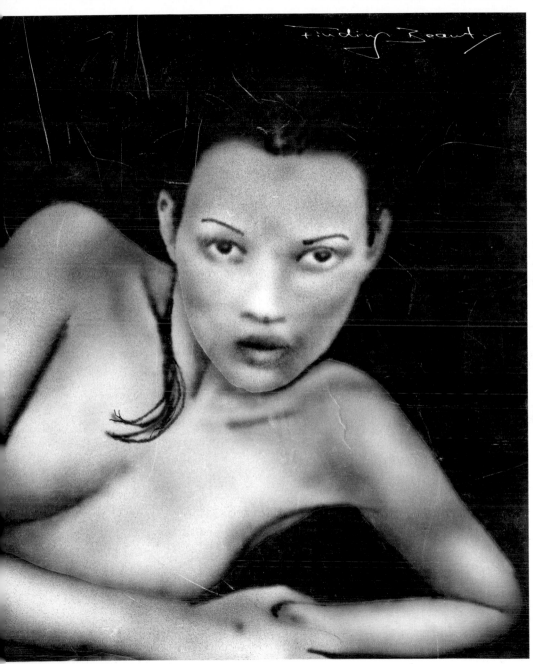

Finding Beauty

HEE JIN KANG

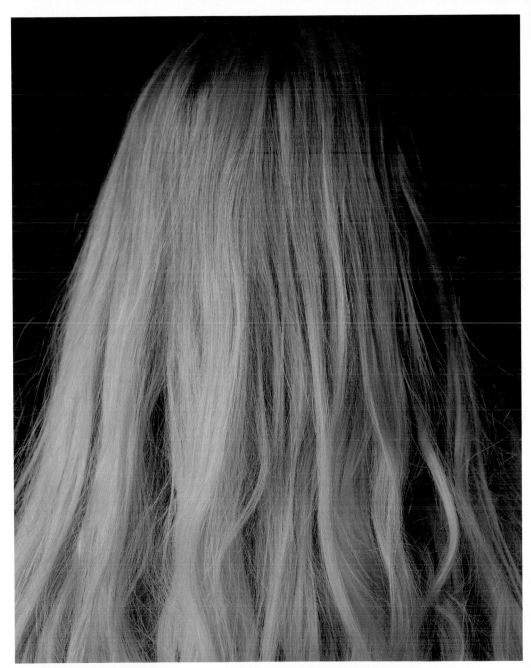

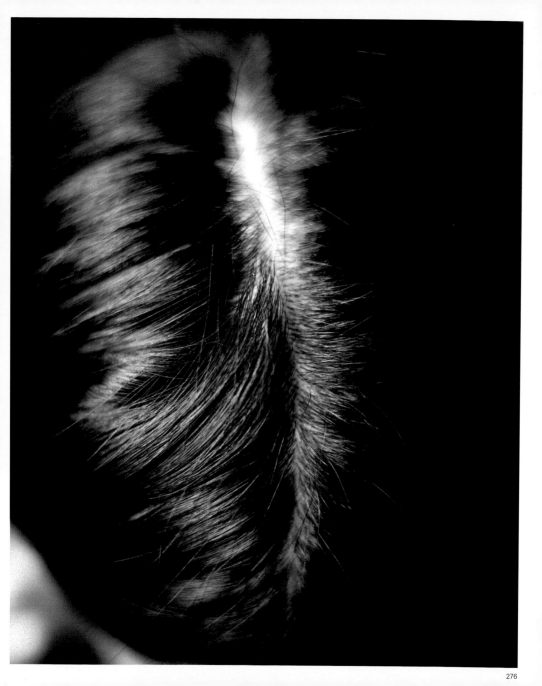

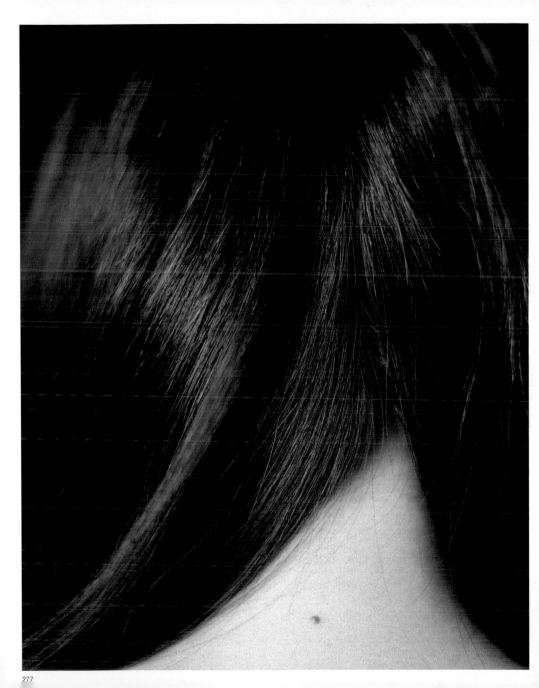

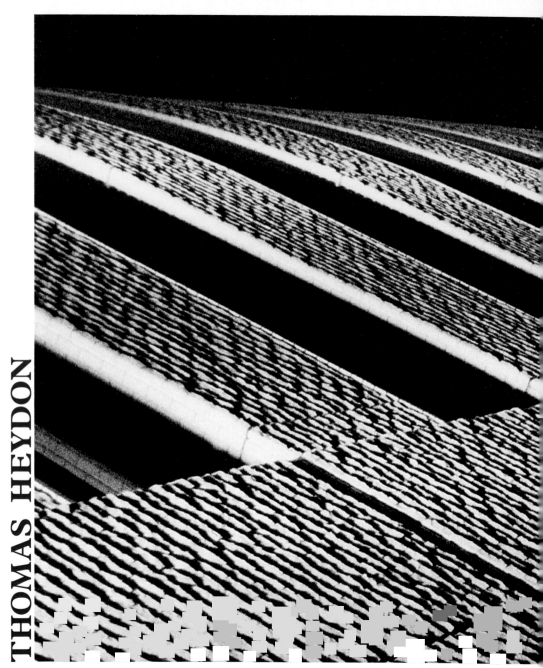

THOMAS HEYDON

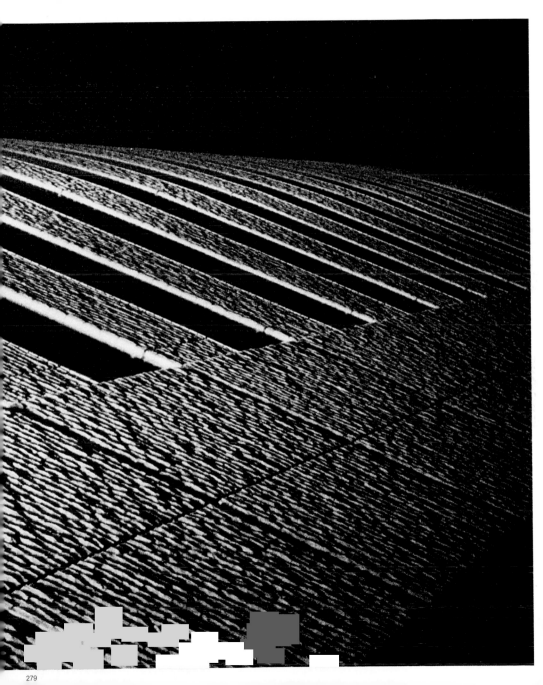

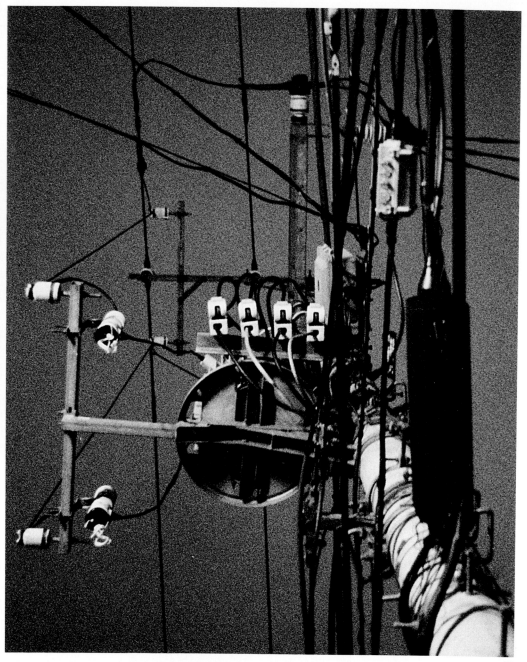

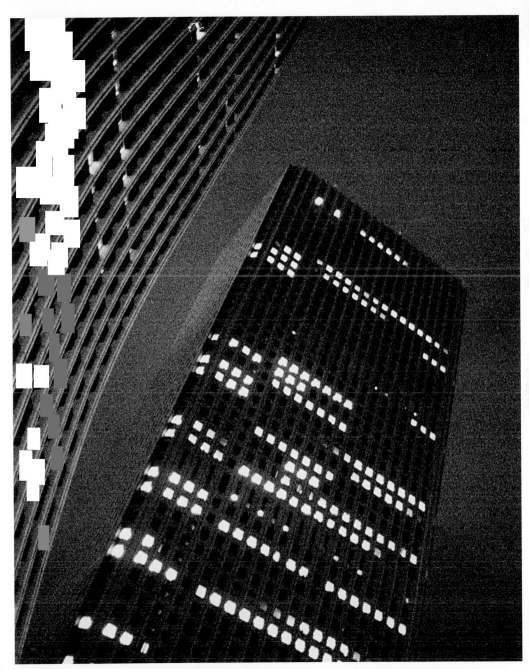

KHOSROW HASSANZADEH

courtesy Rose Issa

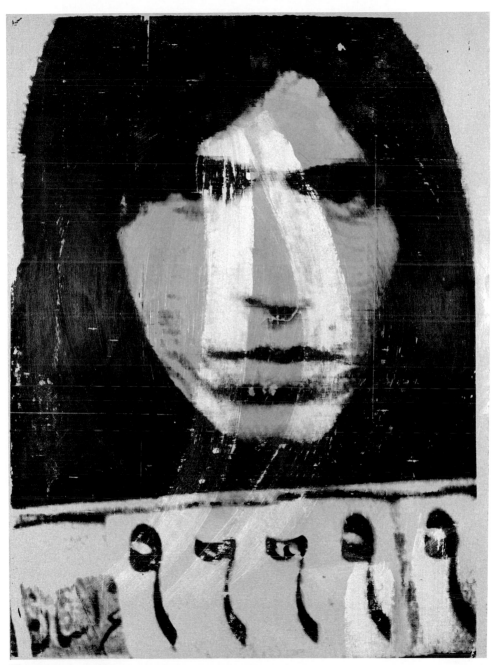

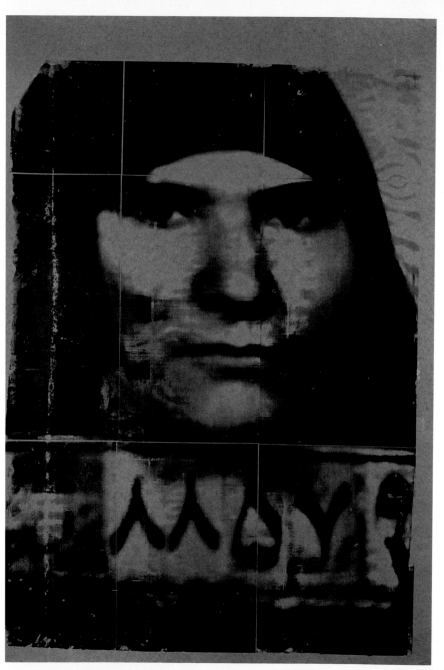

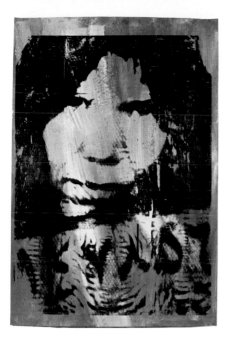
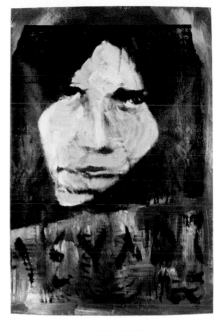
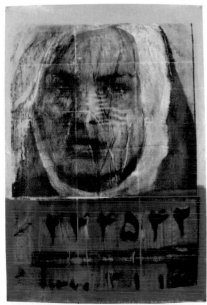
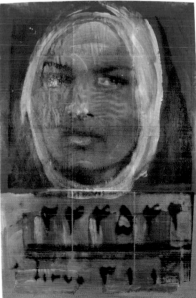

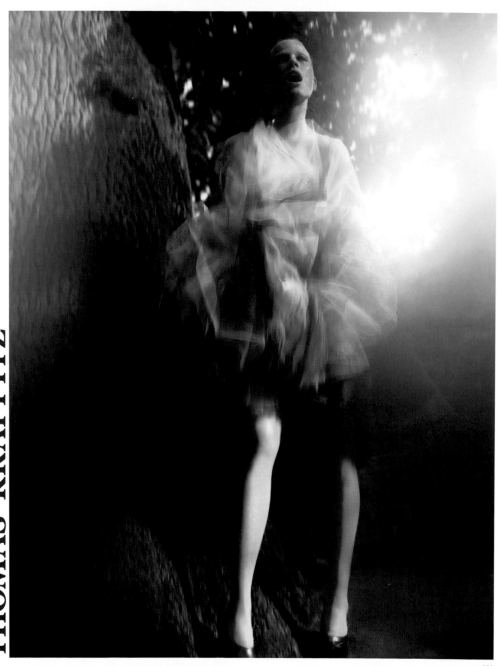

THOMAS KRAPPITZ

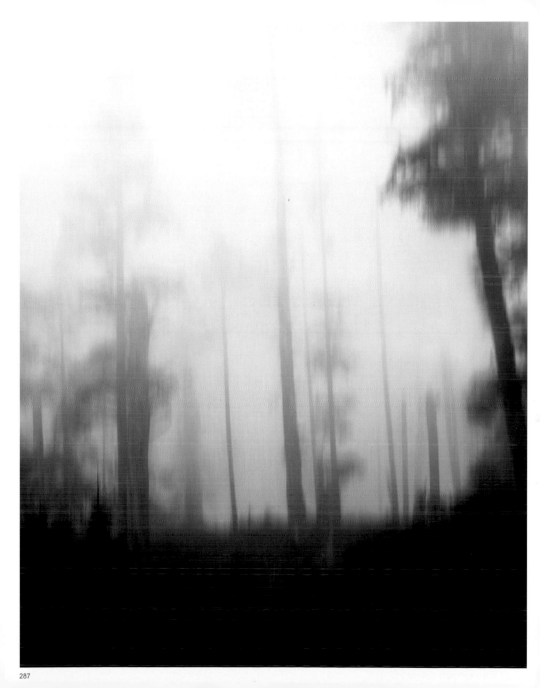

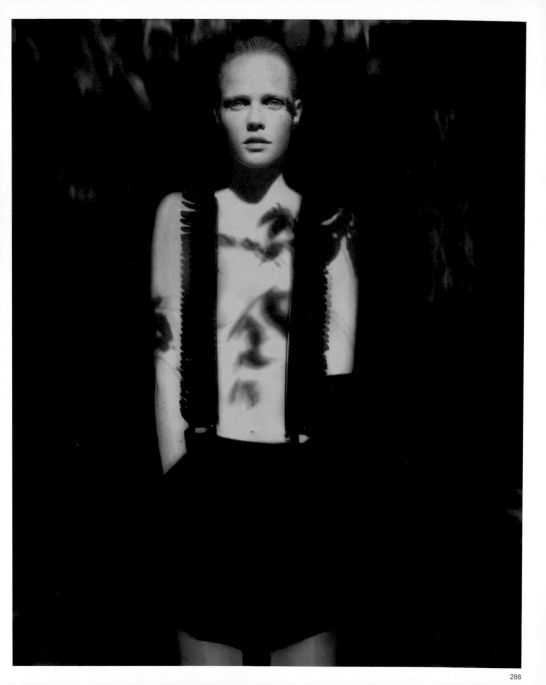

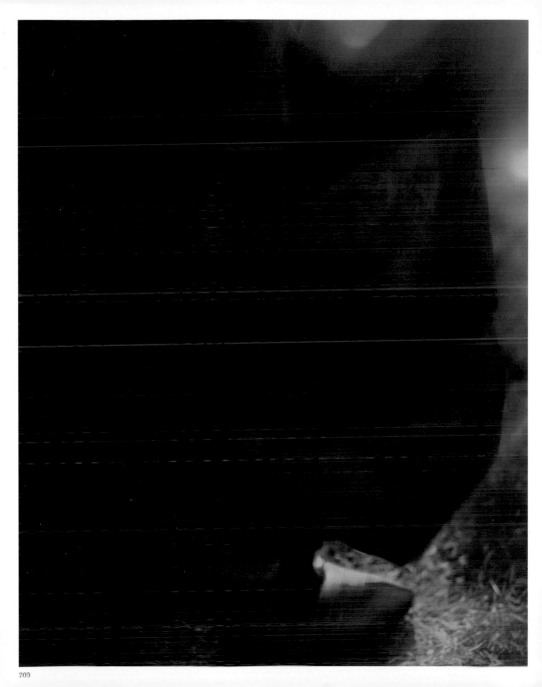

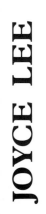

JOYCE LEE

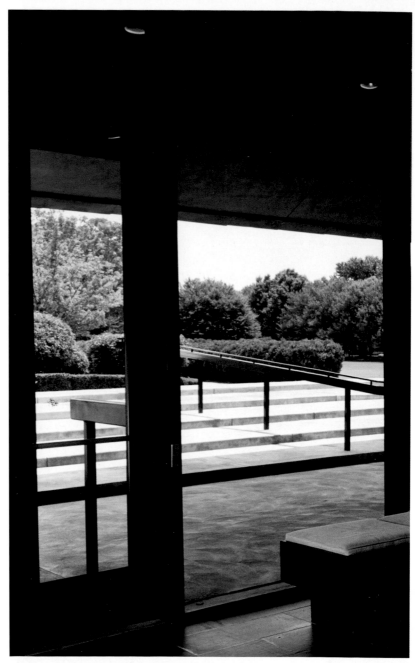

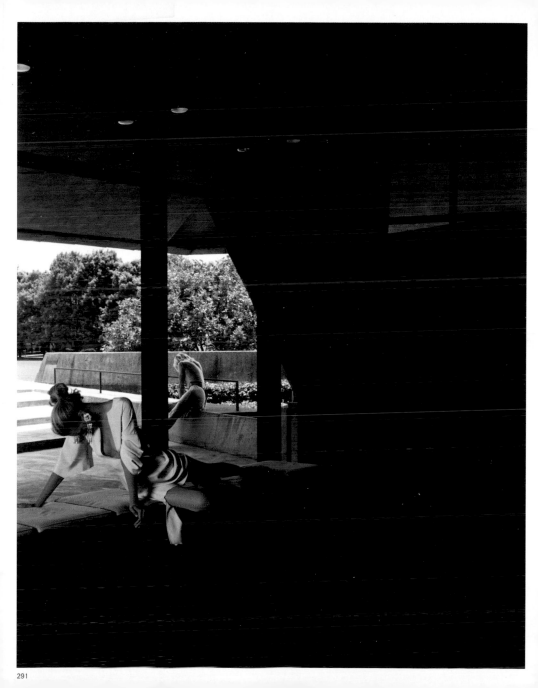

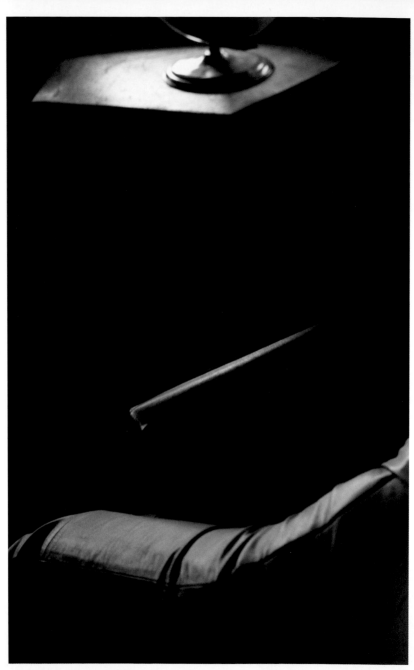

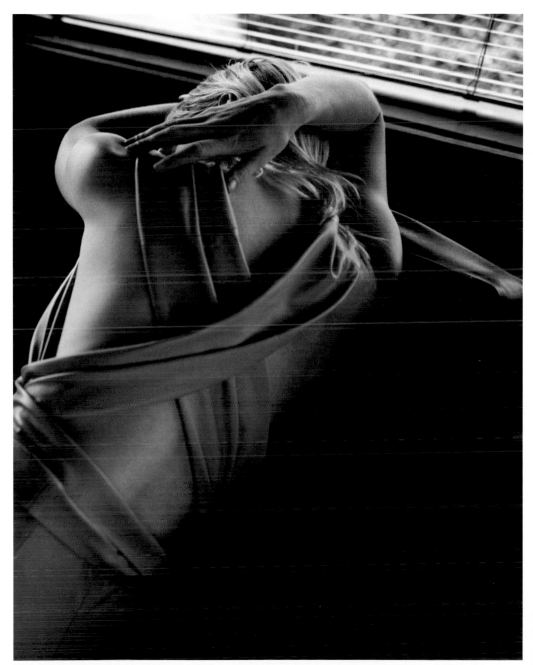

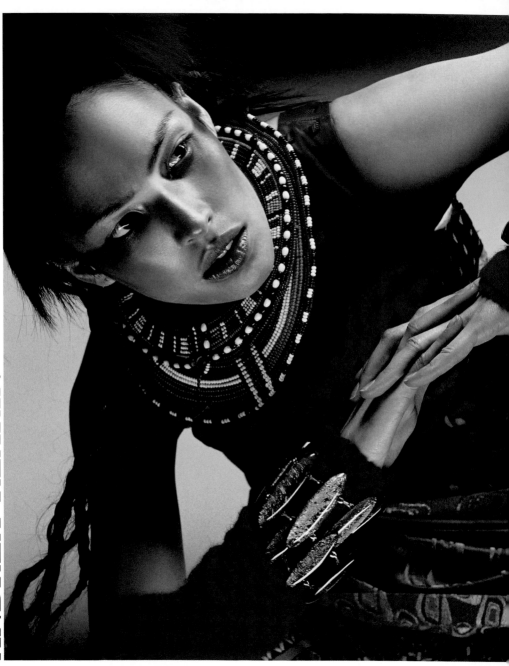

ANDREA KLARIN

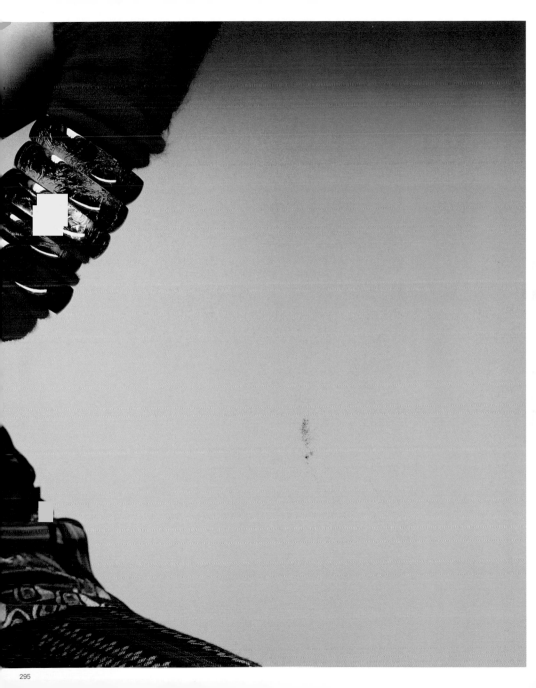

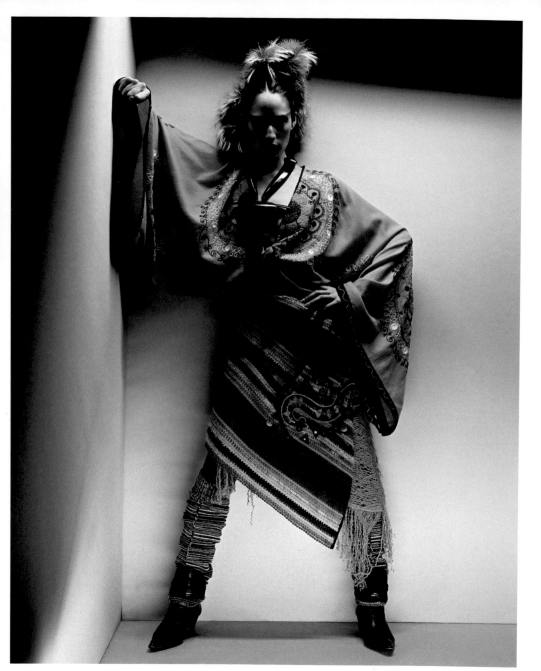

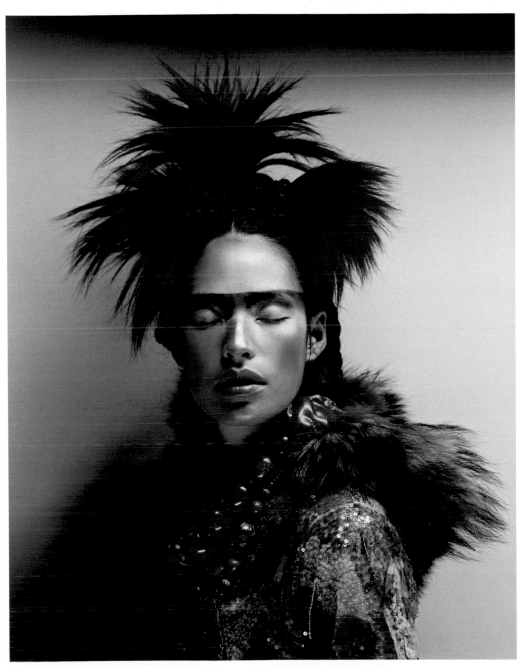

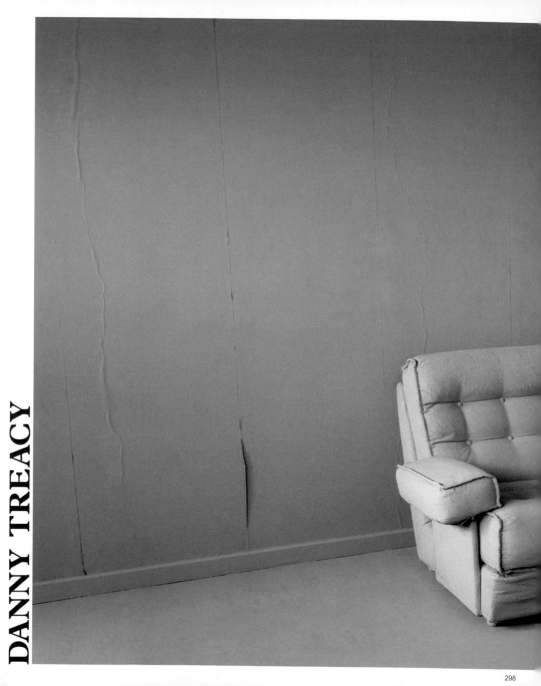

DANNY TREACY

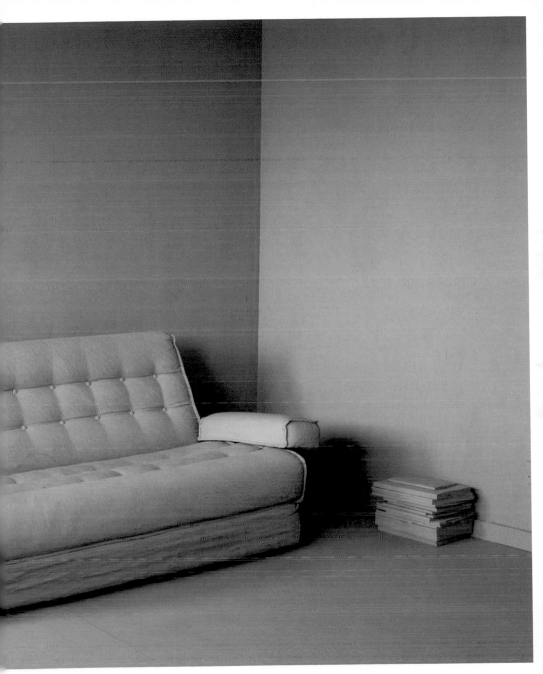

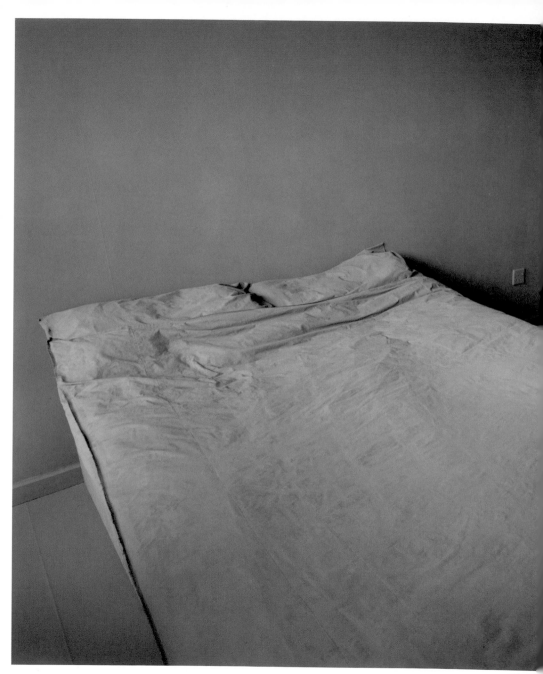

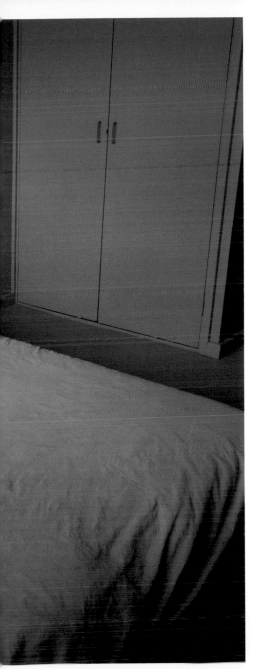

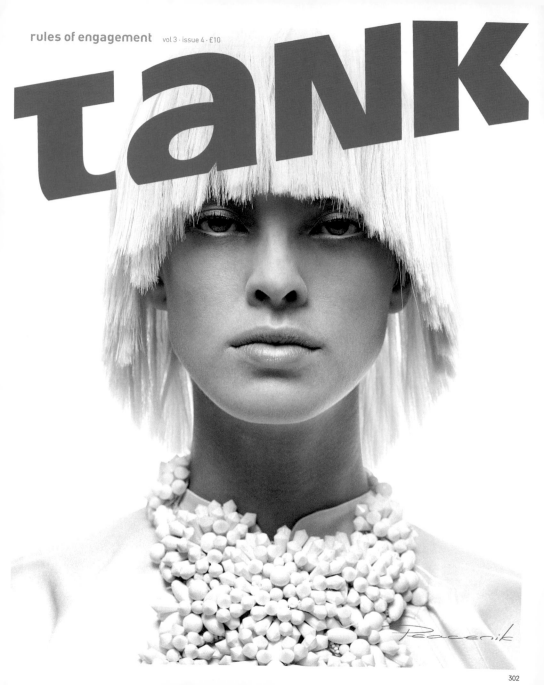

Peacenik

JUST ETIQUETTE

VOLUME 3 · ISSUE 4 · DECEMBER 2002 · COVER PHOTOGRAPH BY GREG LOTUS

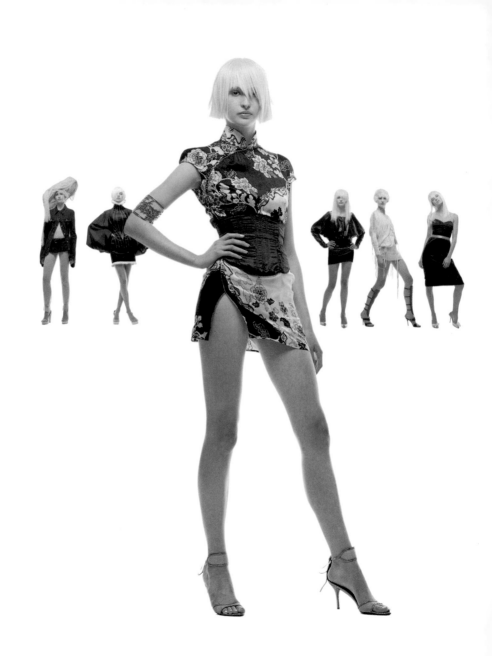

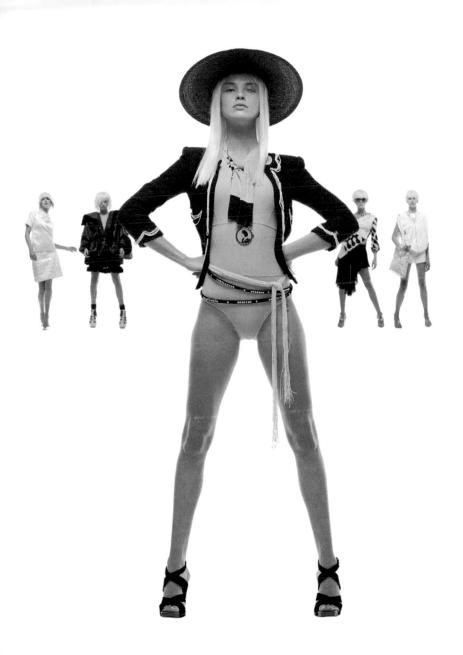

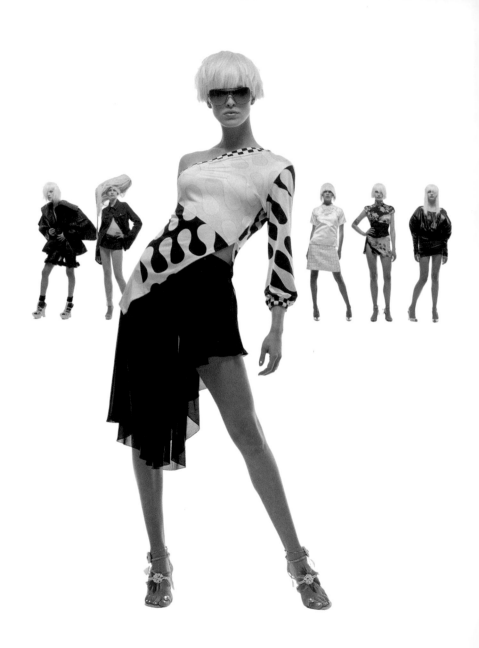

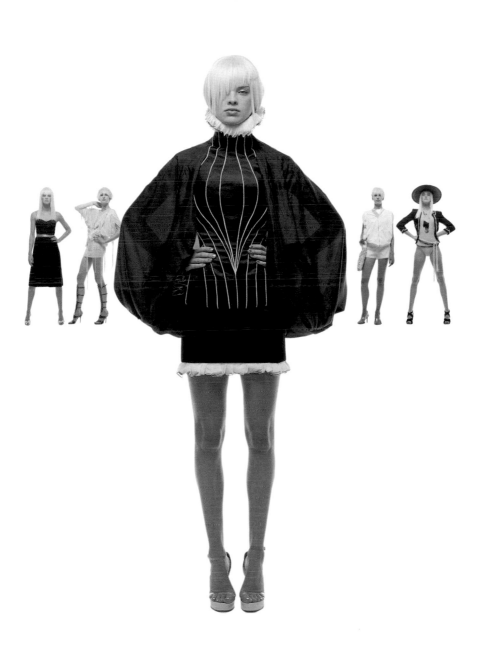

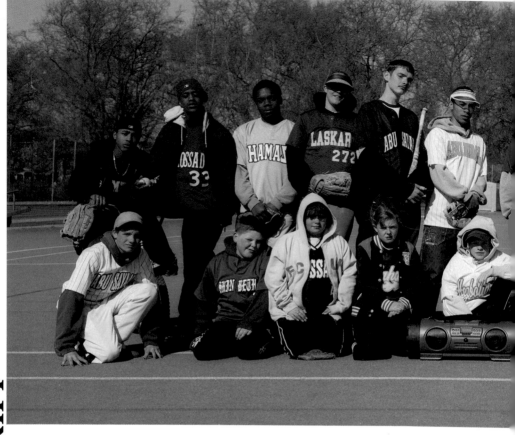

PAYAM SHARIFI

photographs by Alan Clarke

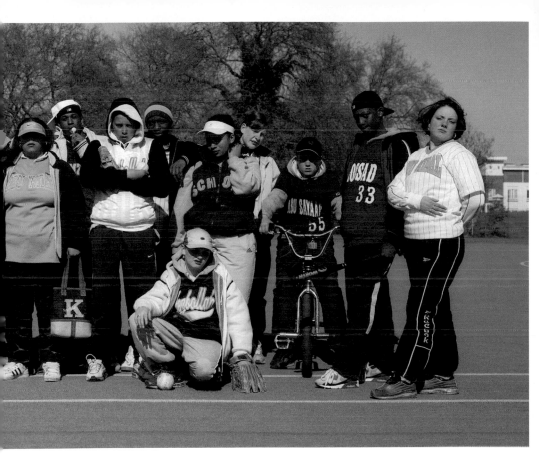

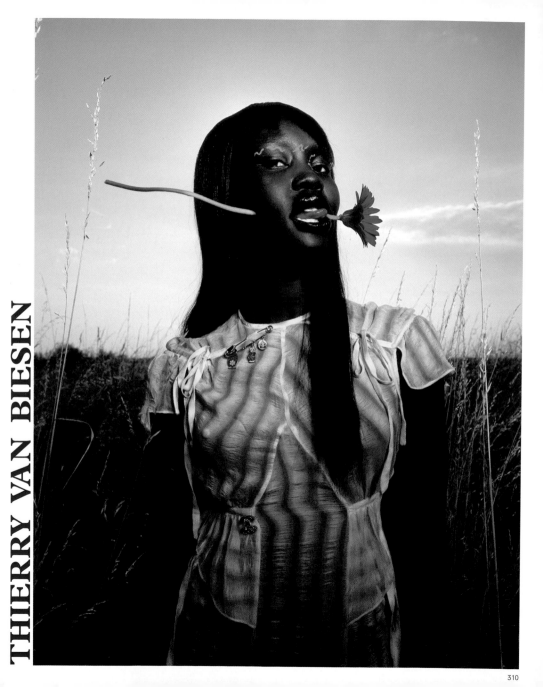

THIERRY VAN BIESEN

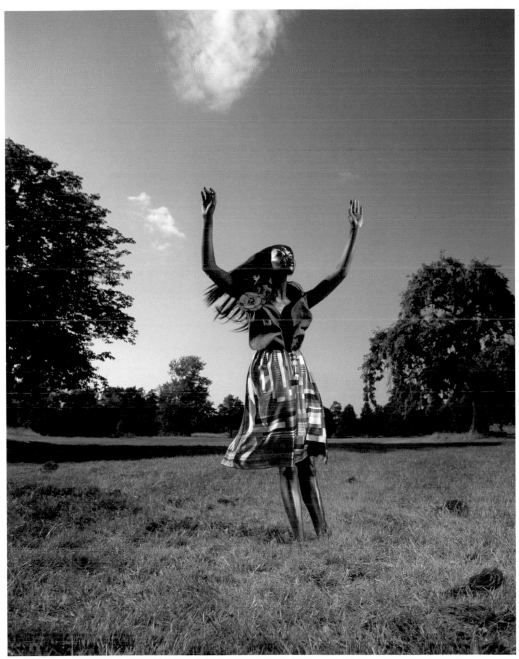

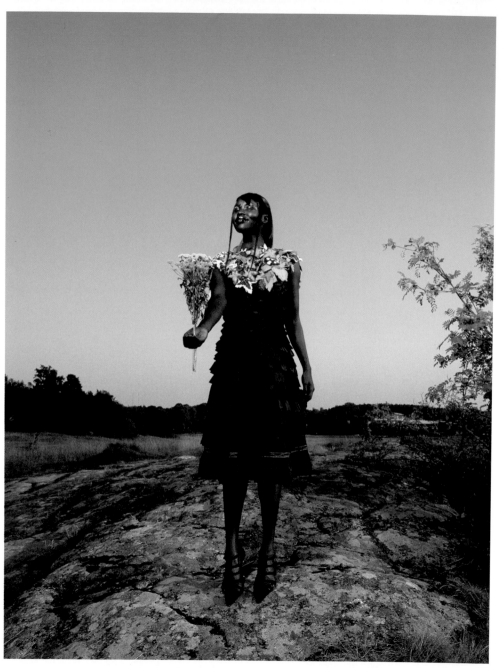

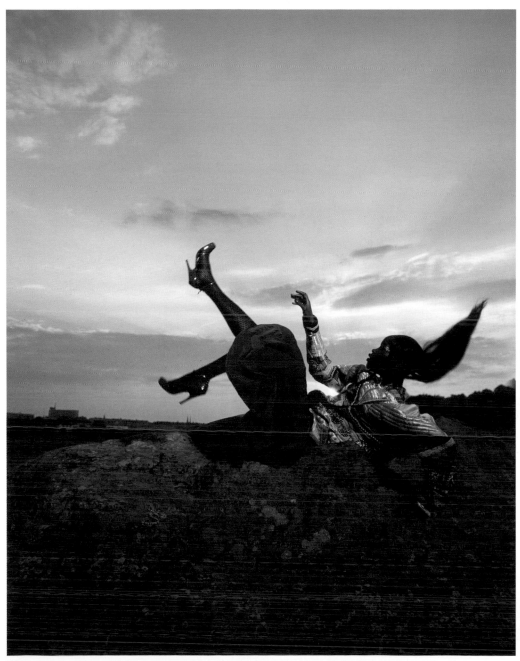

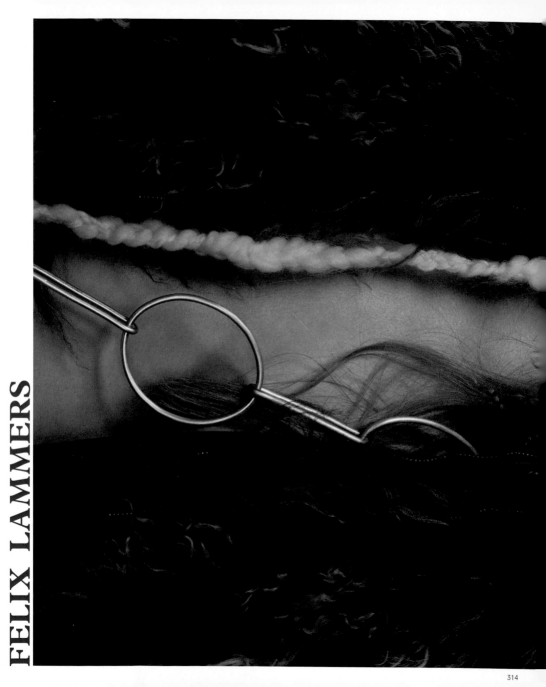

FELIX LAMMERS

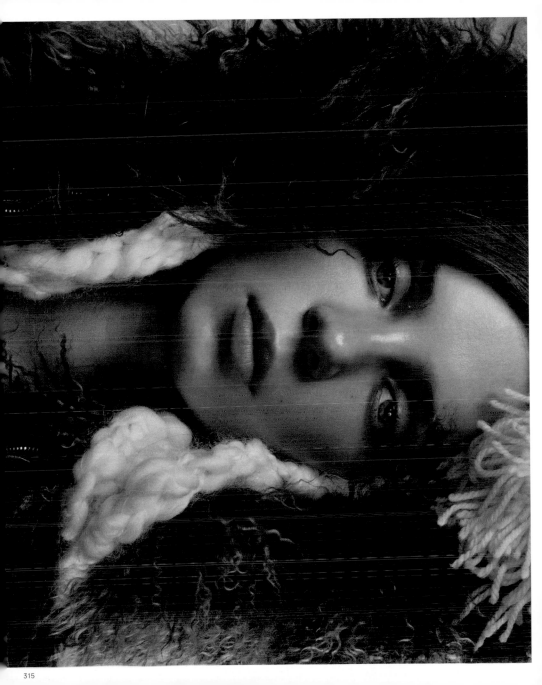

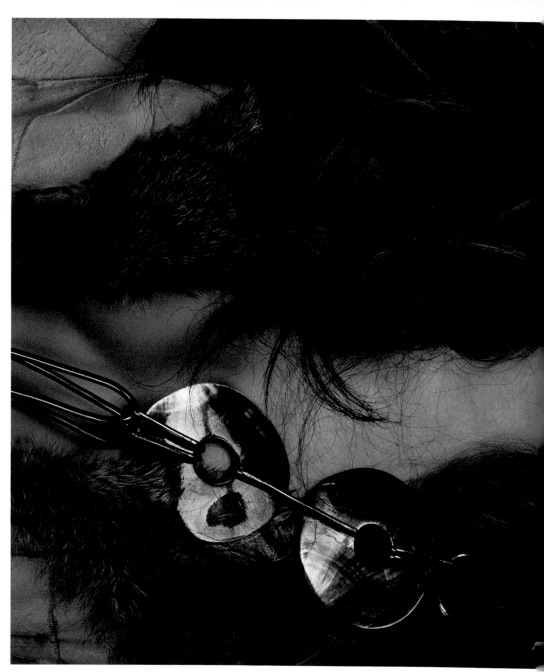

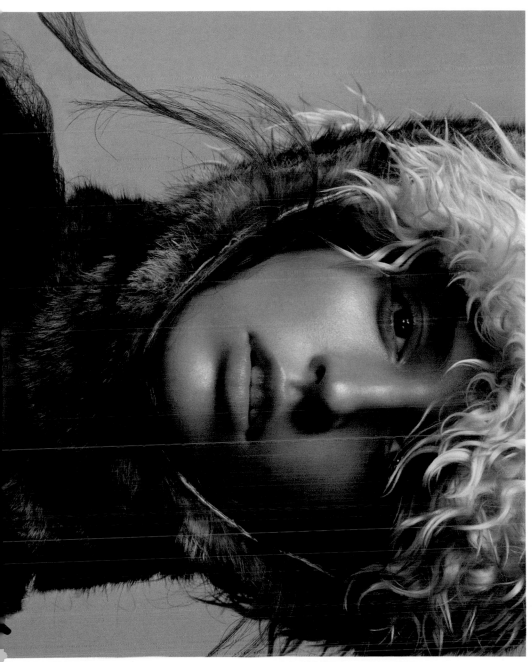

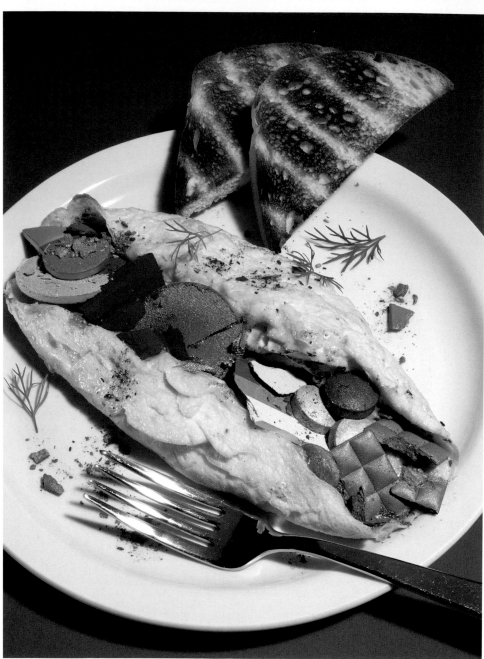

JAMES WOJIK

318

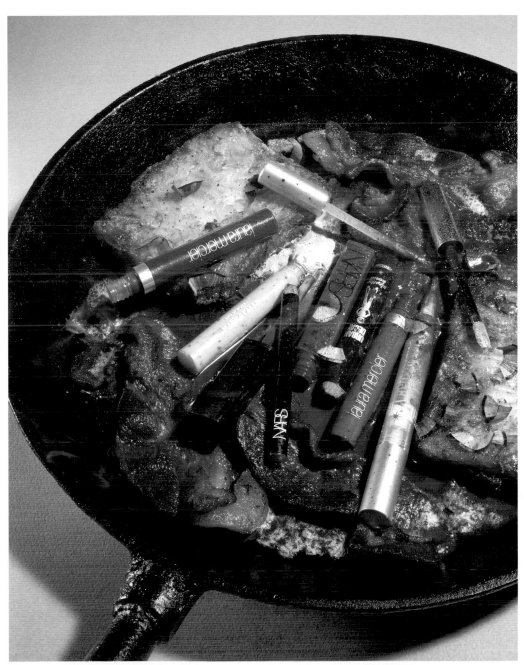

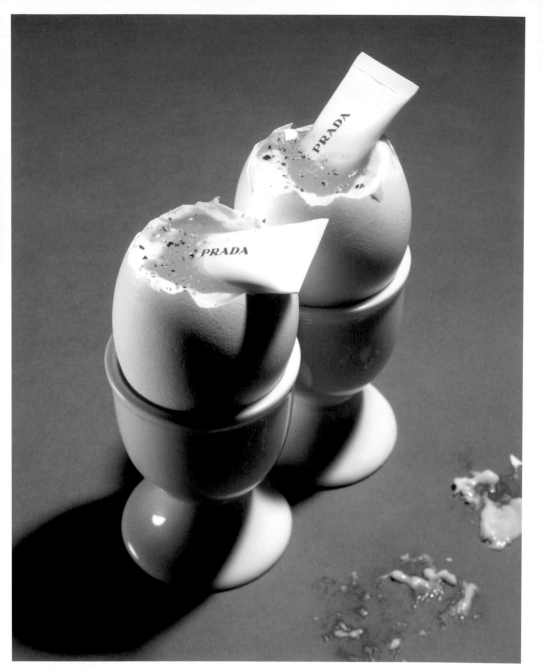

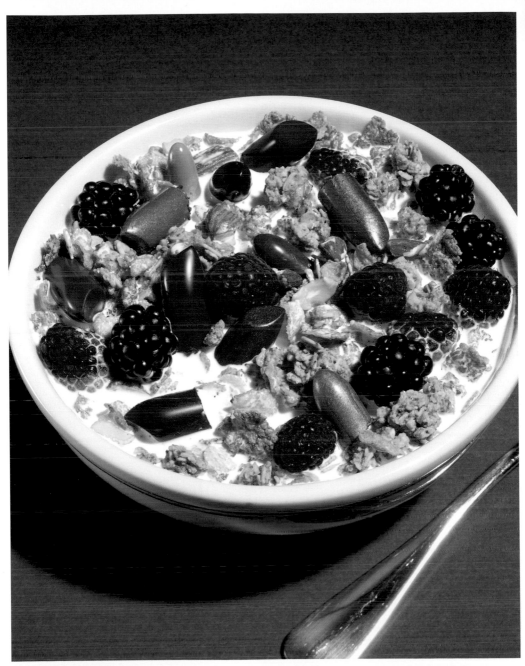

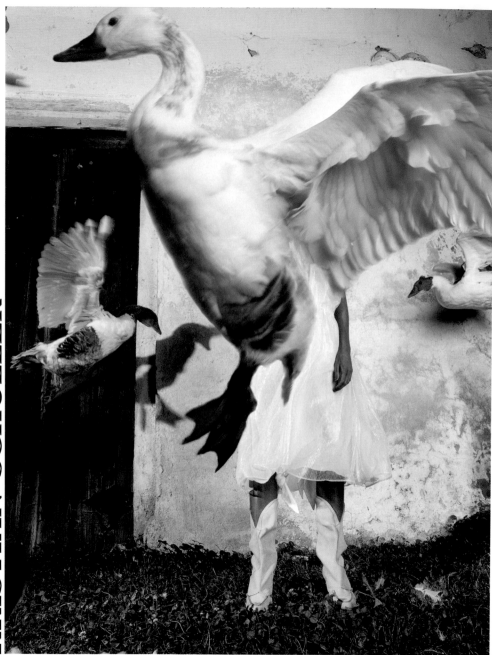

KRISTIAN SCHULLER

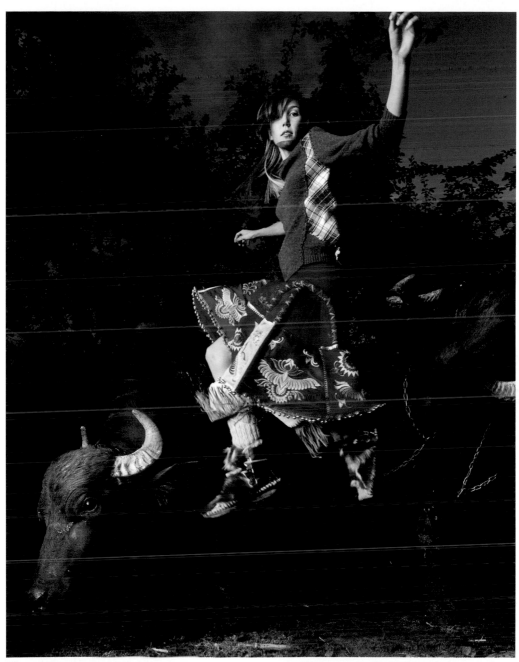

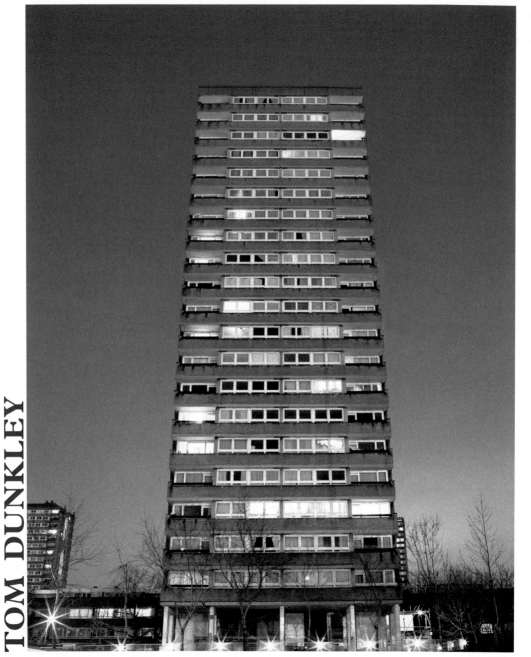

TOM DUNKLEY

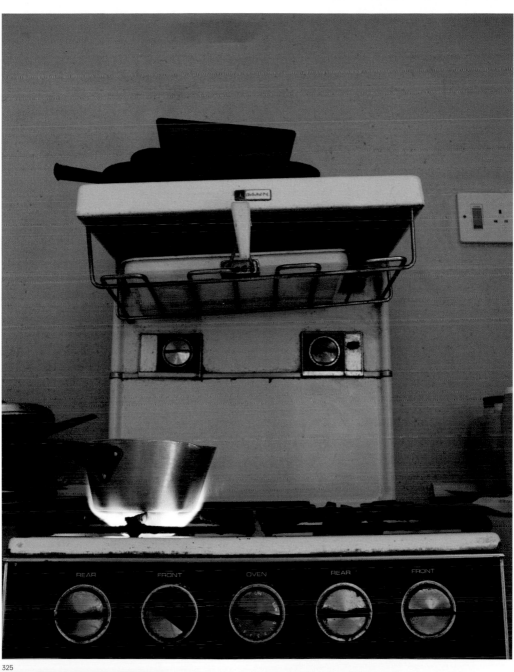

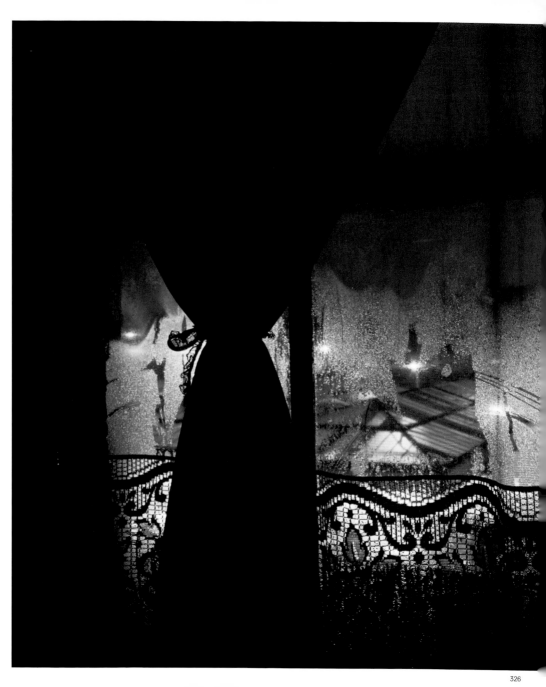

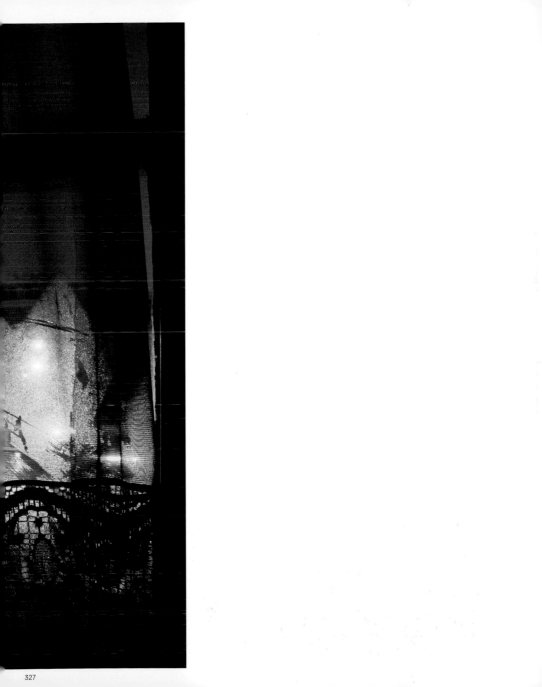

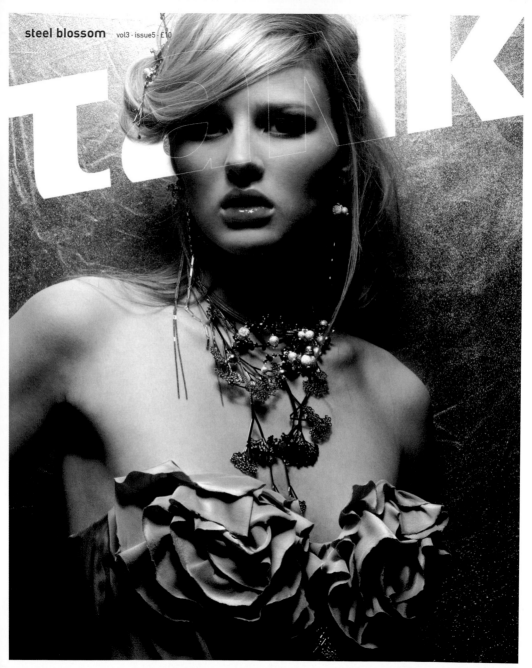

BEAUTY AND RESOLVE

VOLUME 3 · ISSUE 5 · MARCH 2003 · COVER PHOTOGRAPH BY MASOUD

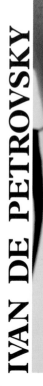

IVAN DE PETROVSKY

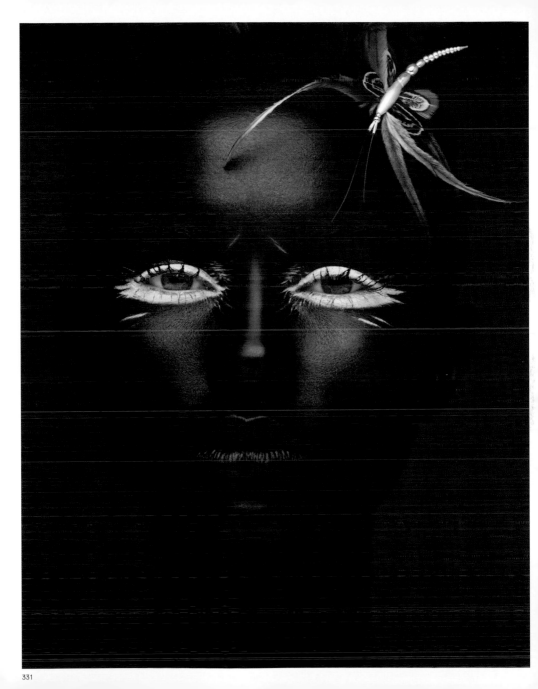

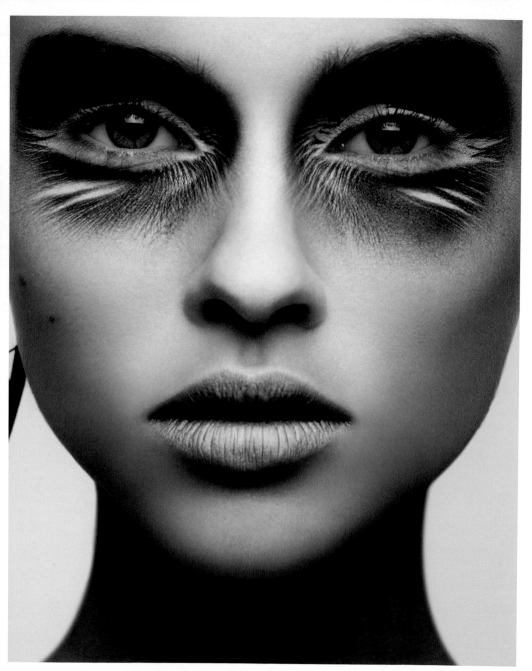

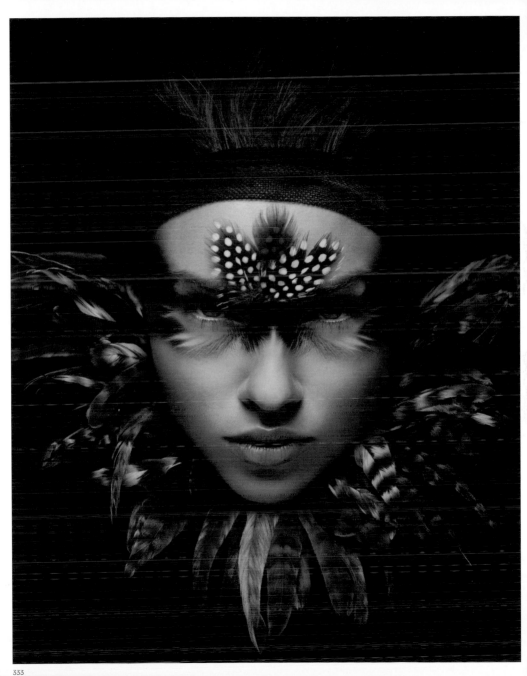

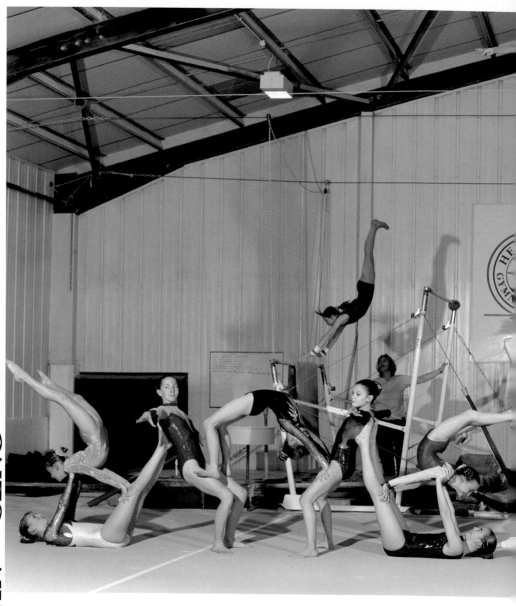

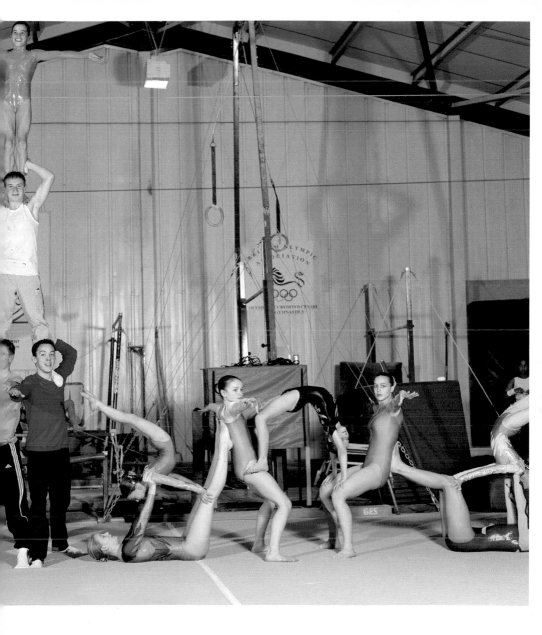

EDGAR MARTINS

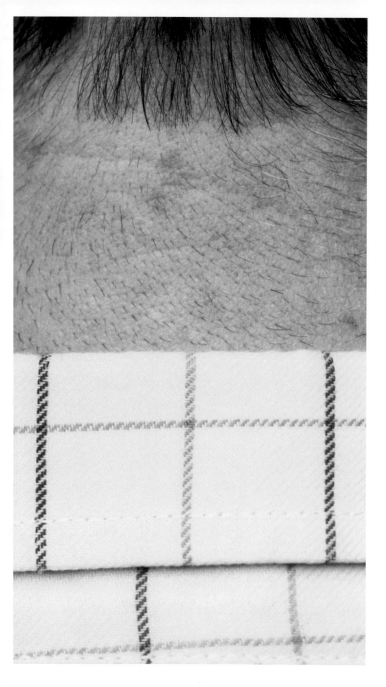

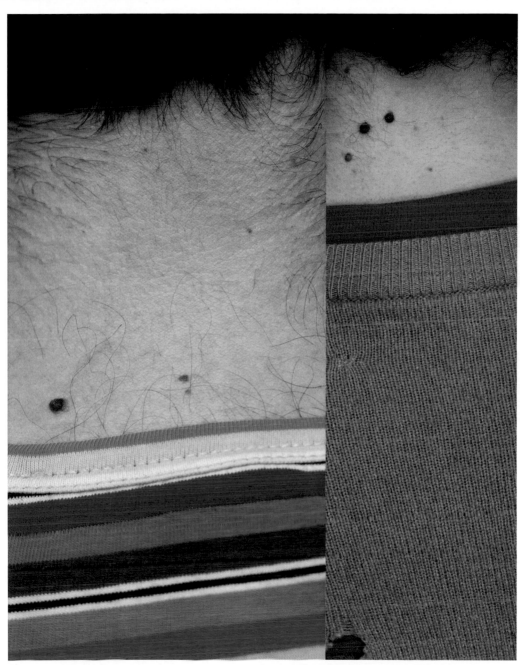

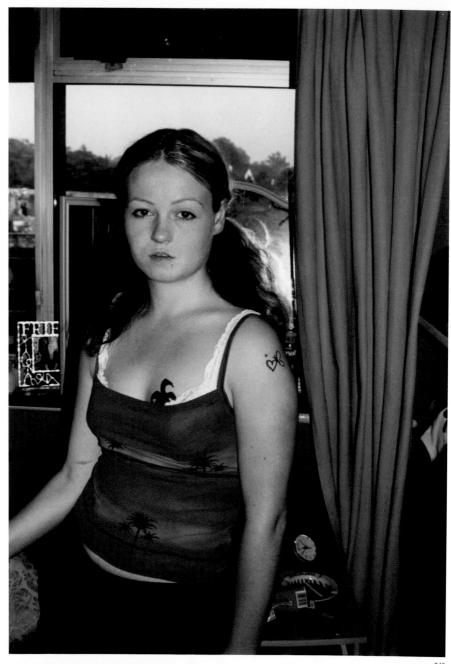
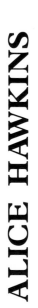

ALICE HAWKINS

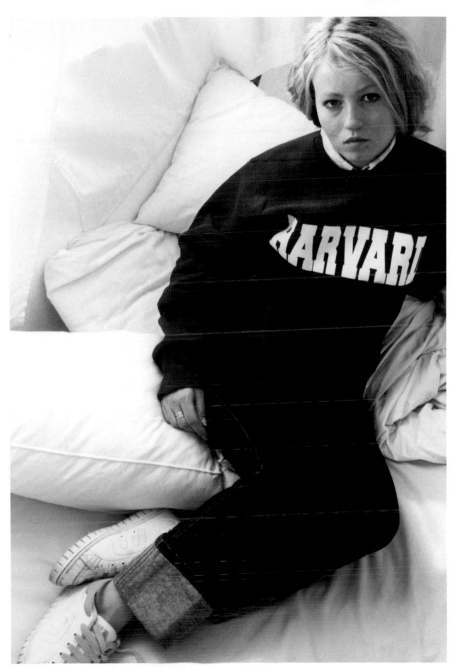

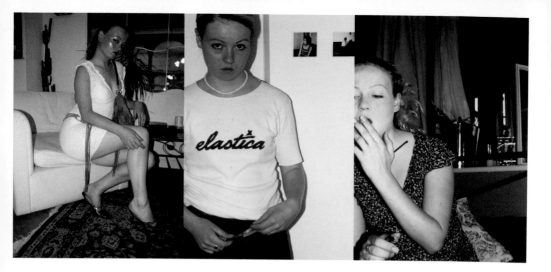

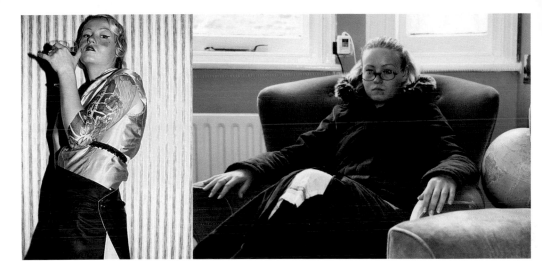

MARK ALESKY

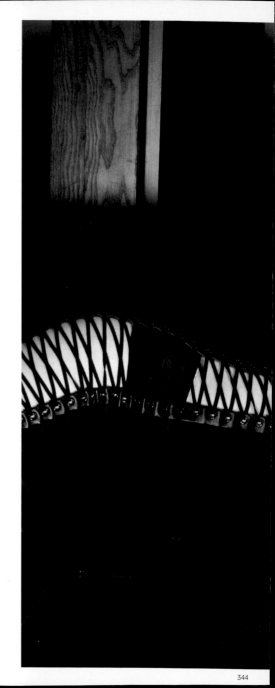

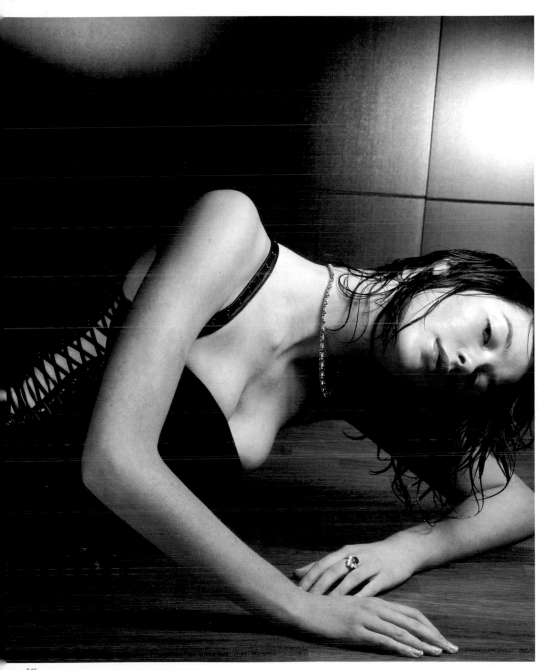

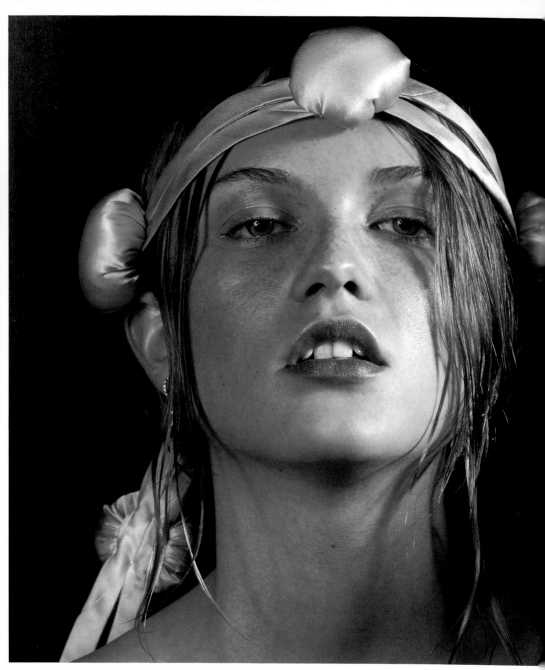

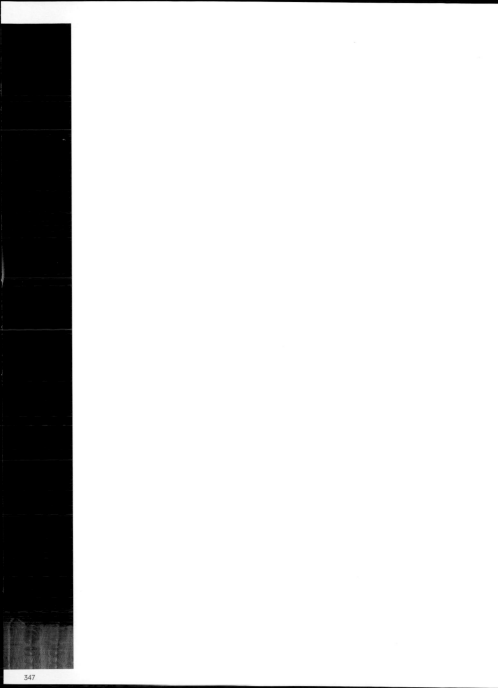

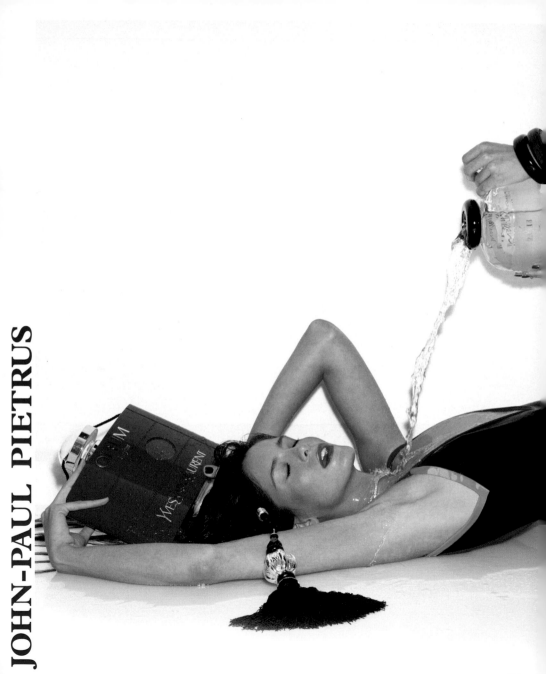

JOHN-PAUL PIETRUS

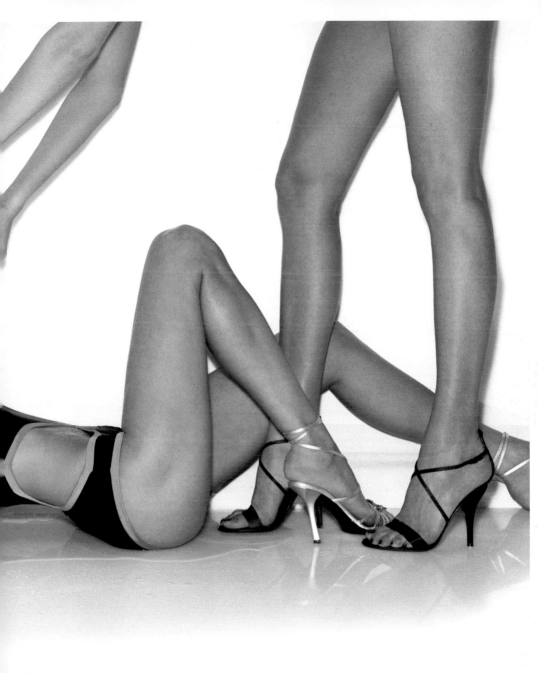

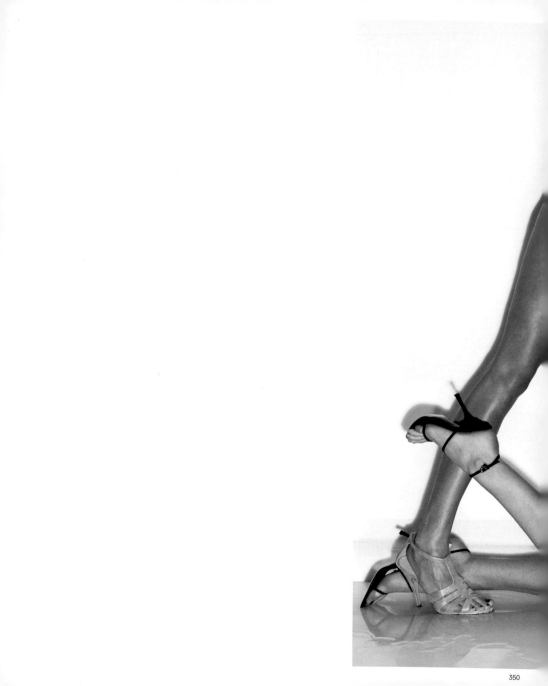

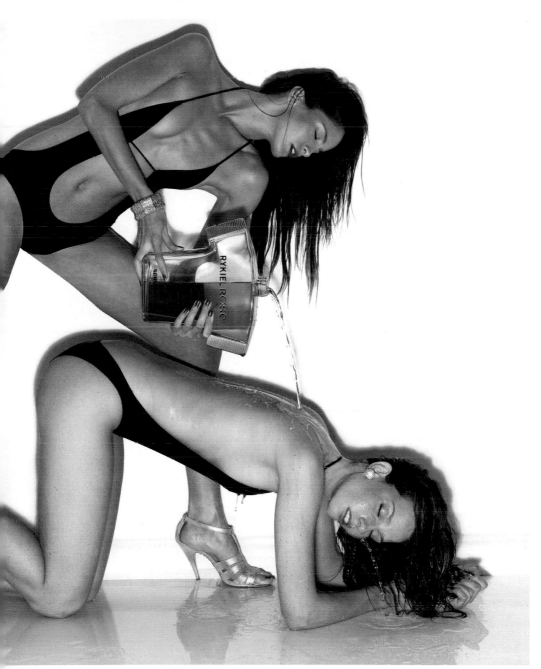

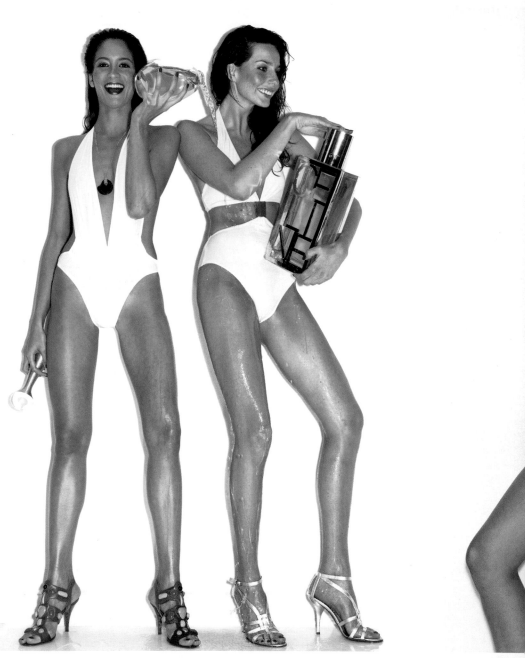

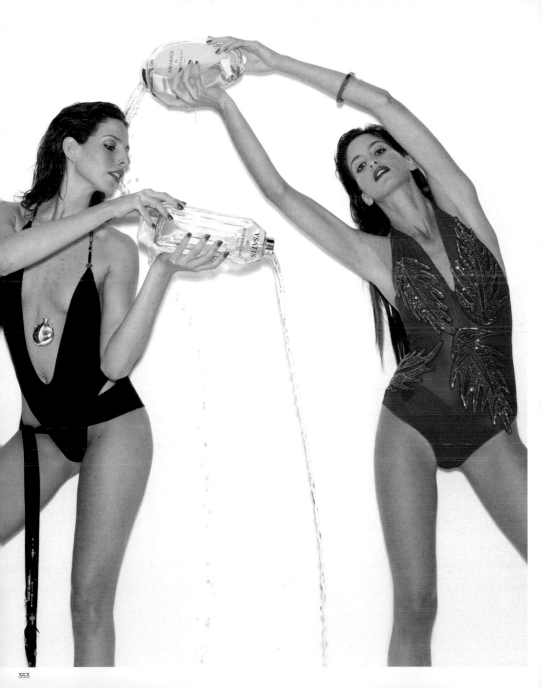

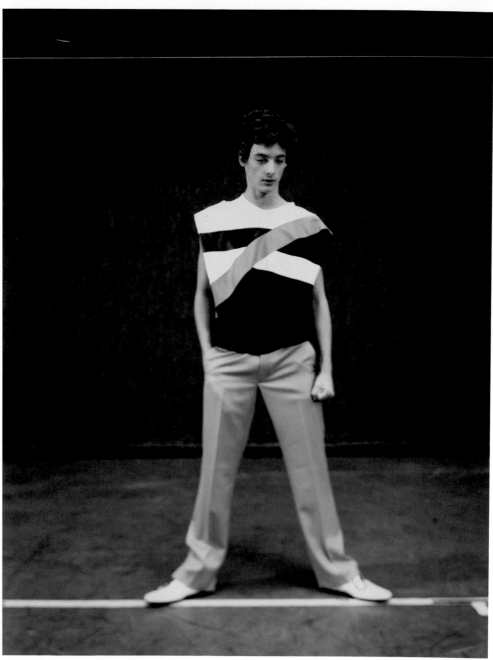

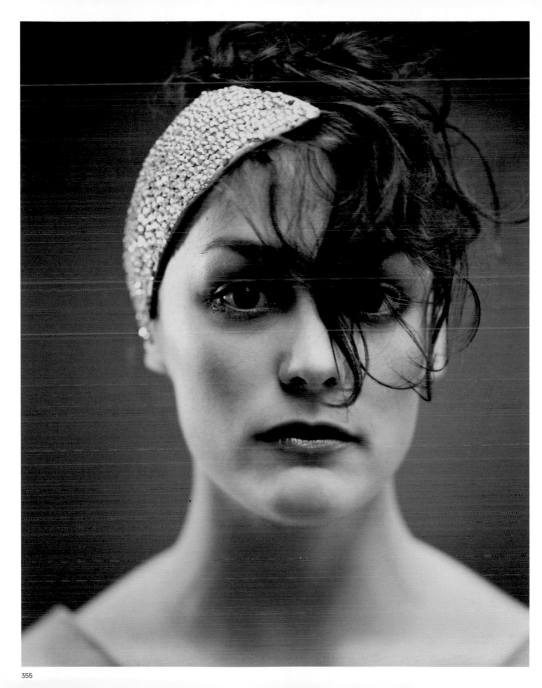

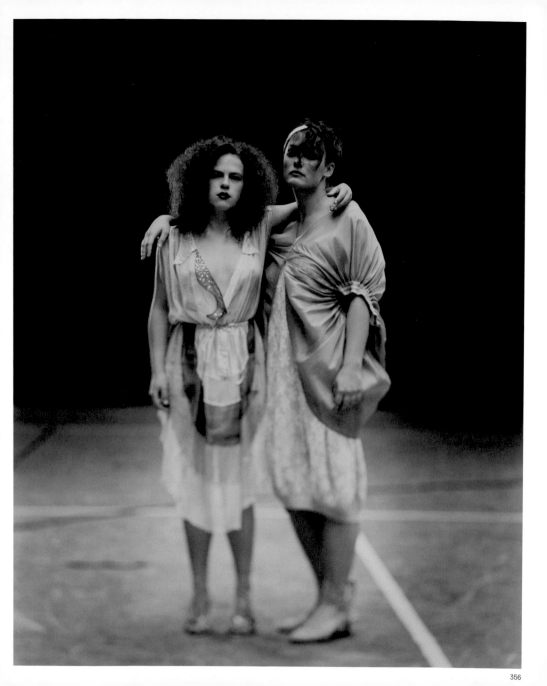

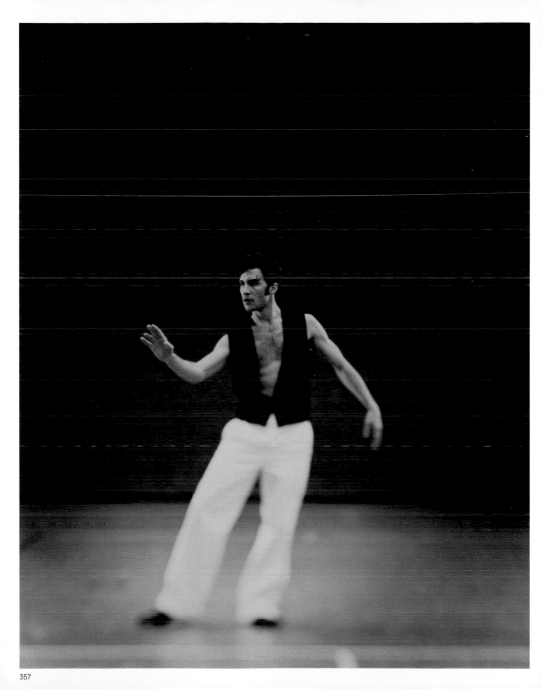

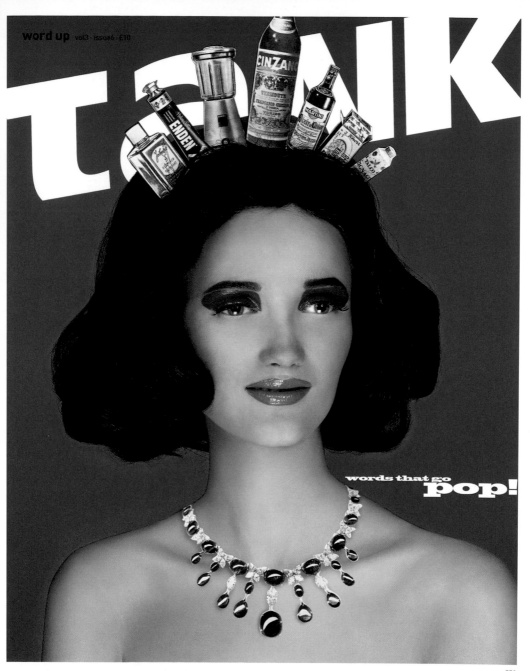

POPULISTA

VOLUME 3 · ISSUE 6 · MAY 2003 · COVER PHOTOGRAPH BY MATTEO BERTOLIO

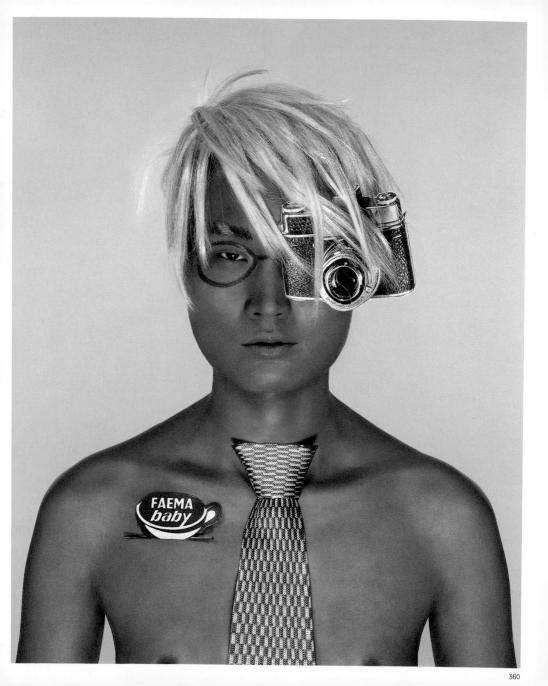

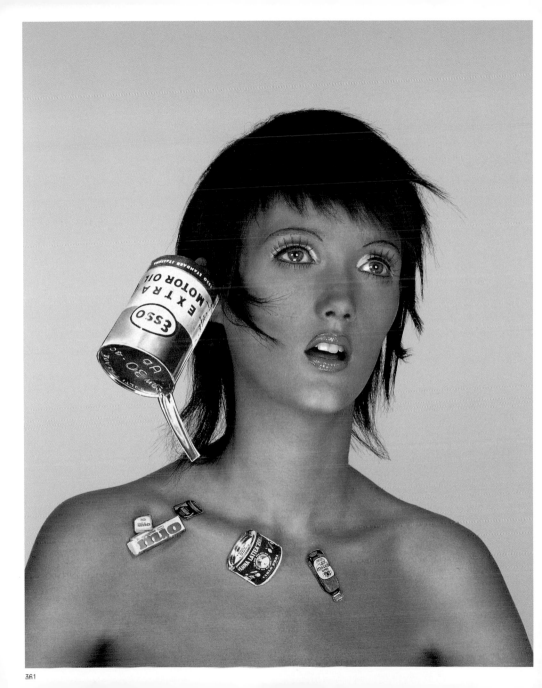

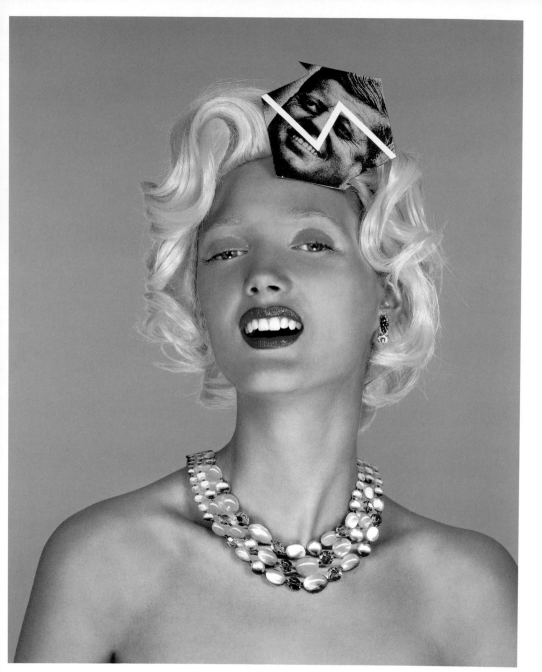

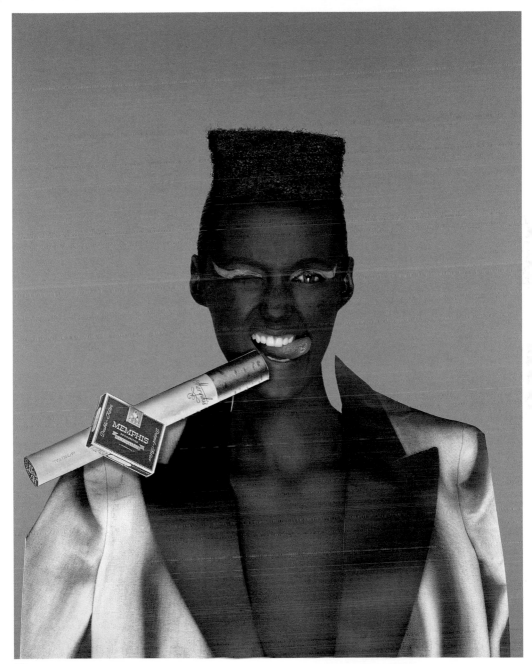

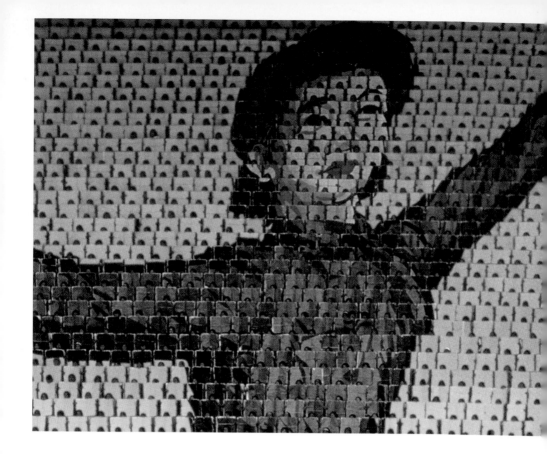

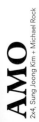

AMO
2x4, Sung Joong Kim + Michael Rock

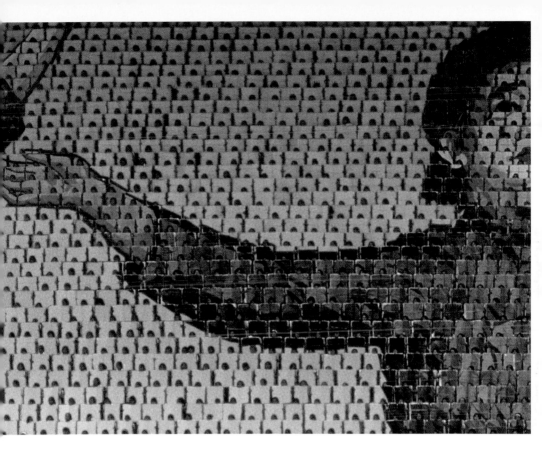

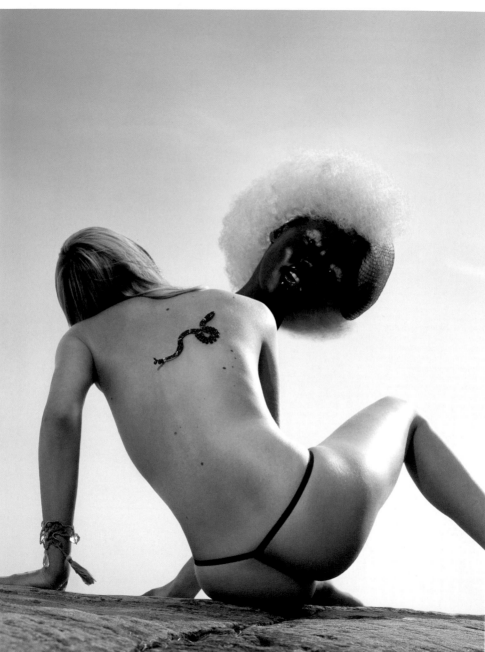

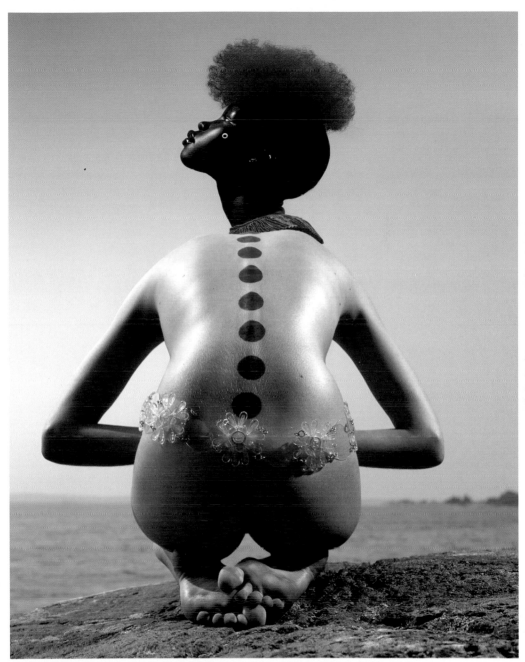

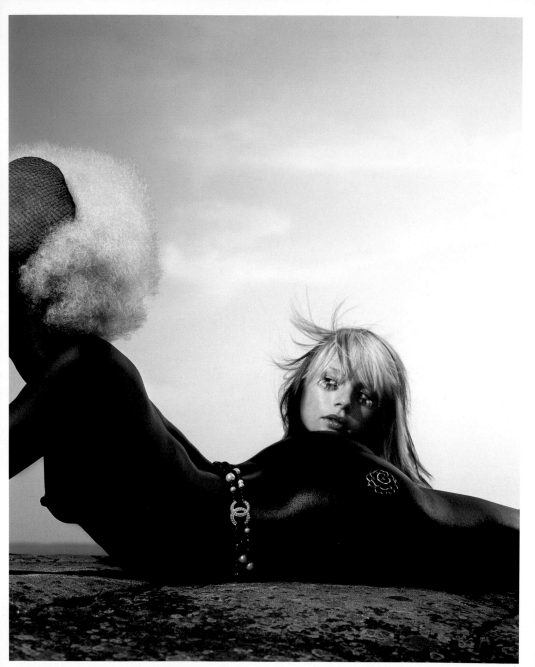

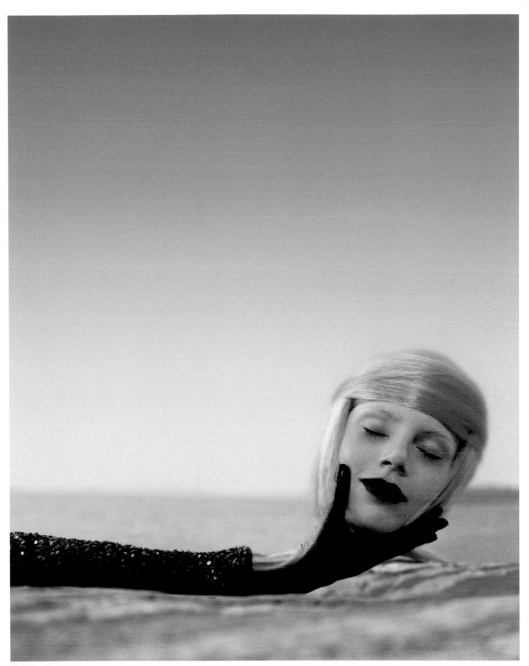

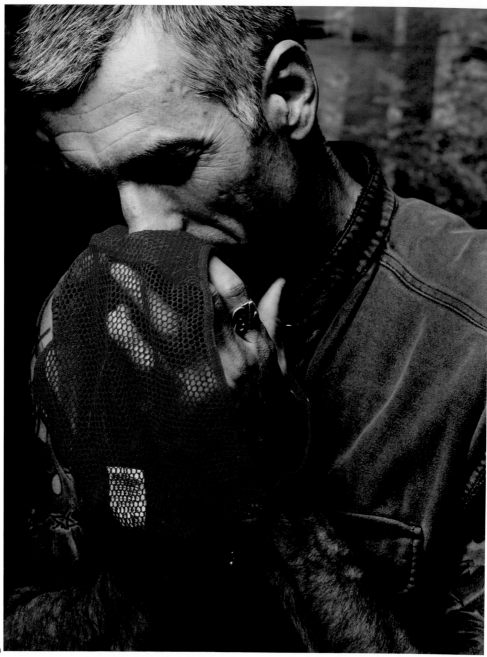

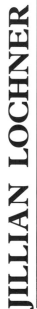

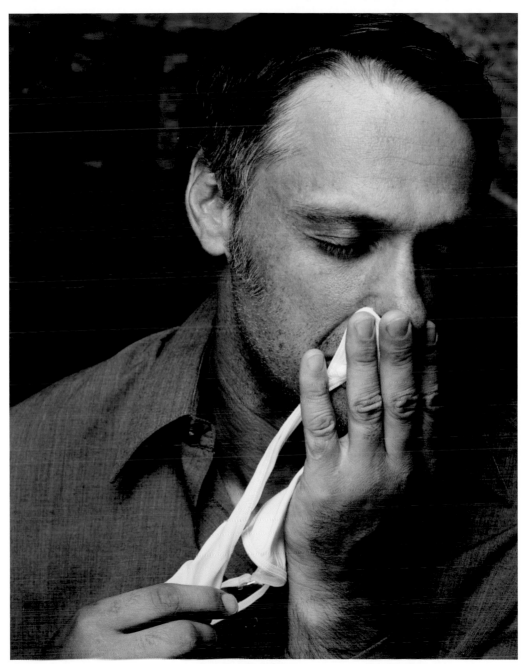

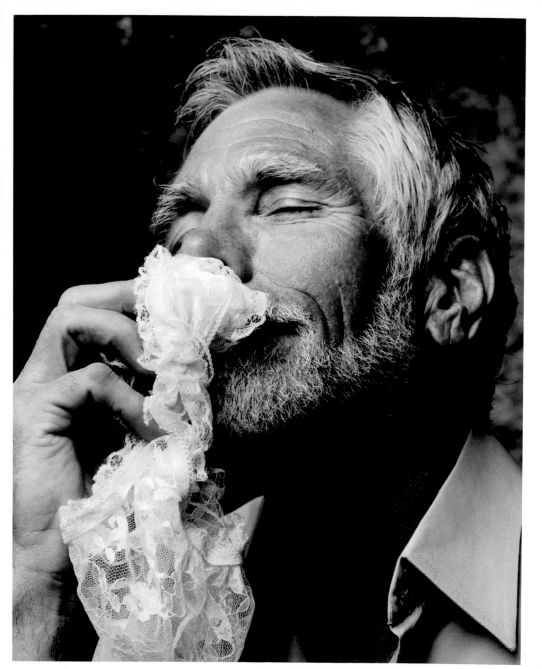

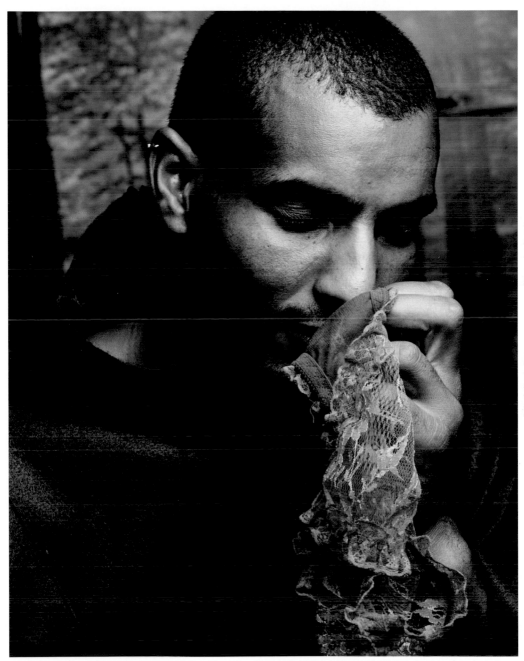

LINNEA LARSSON

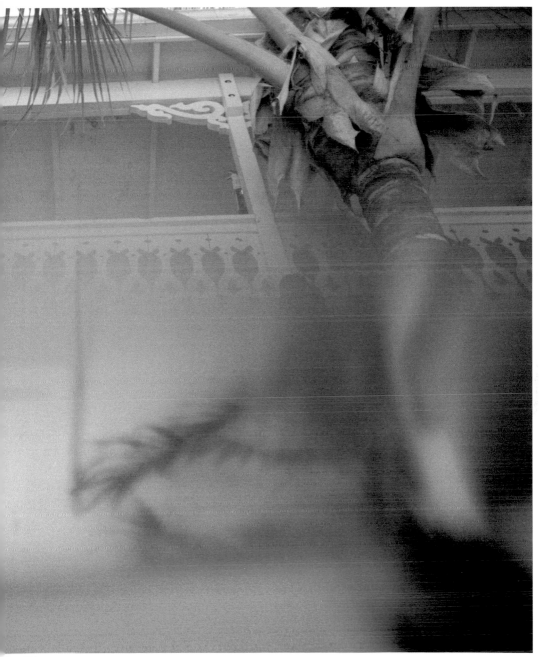

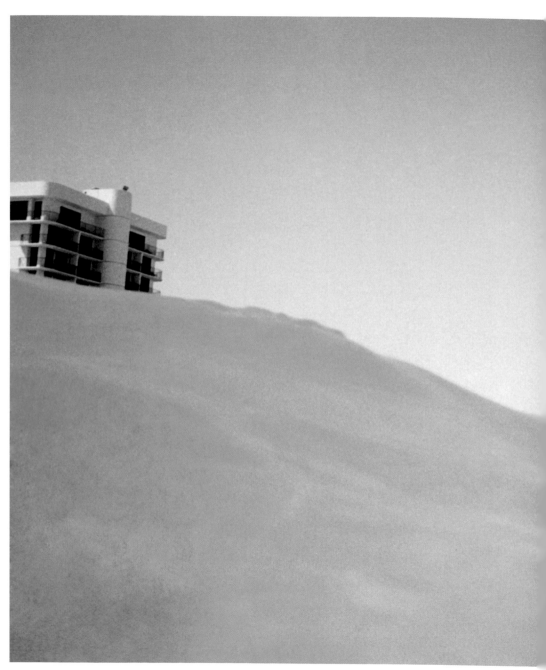

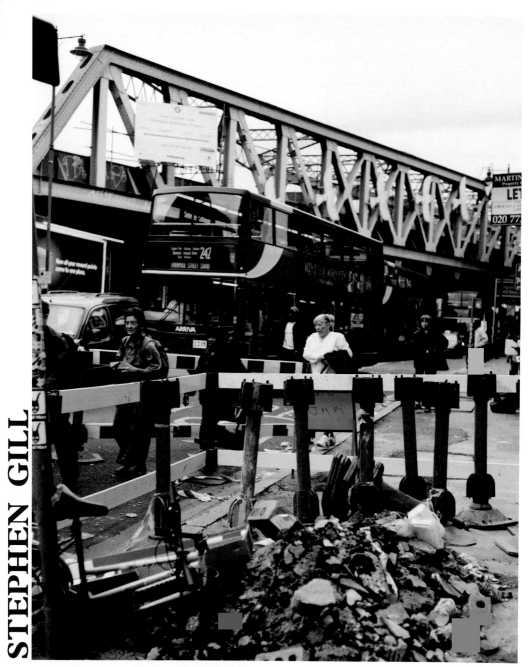

STEPHEN GILL

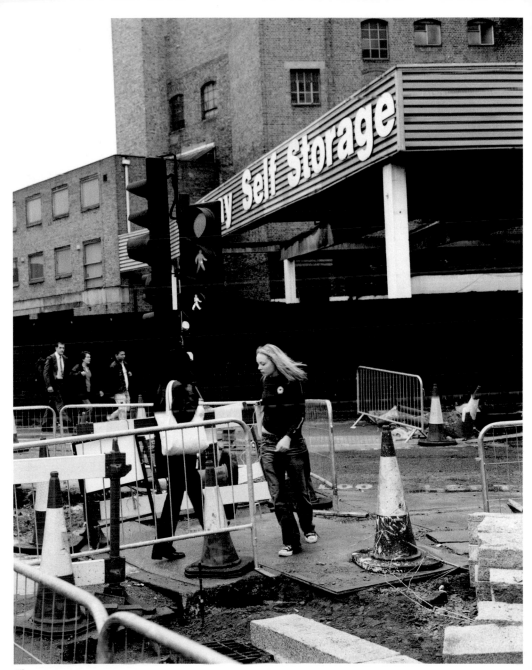

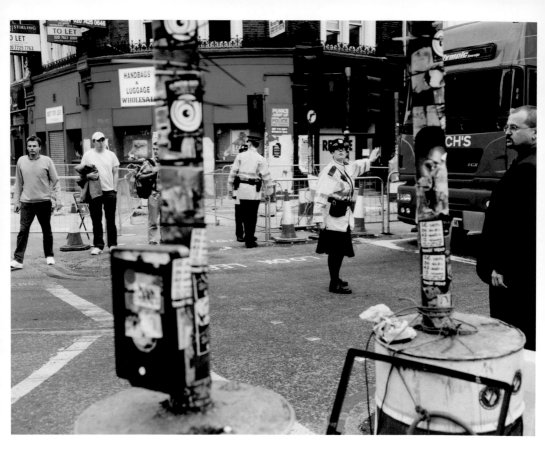

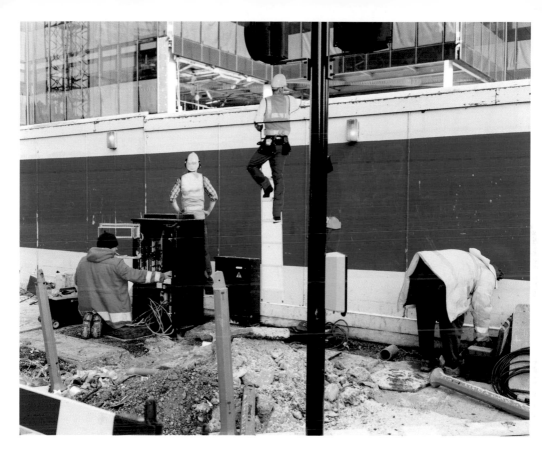

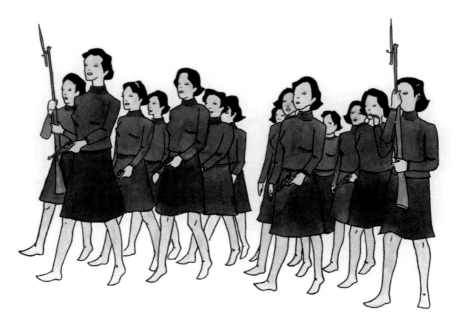

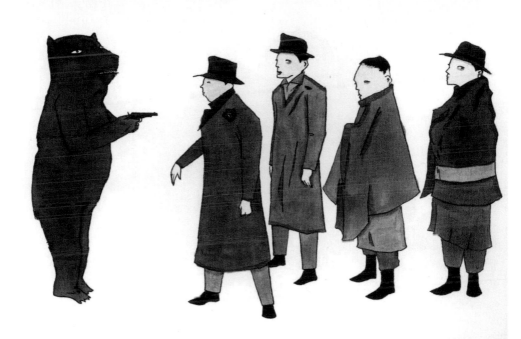

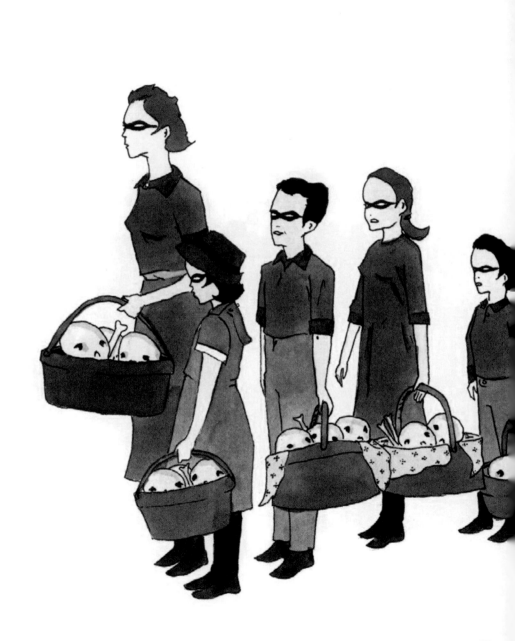

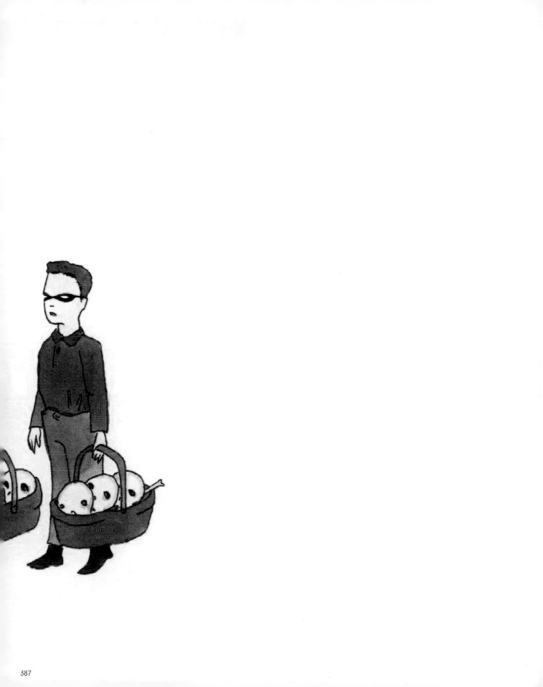

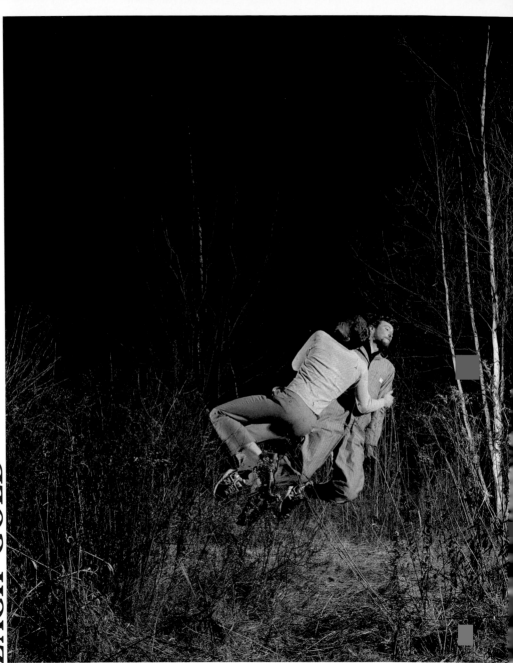

ZACH GOLD

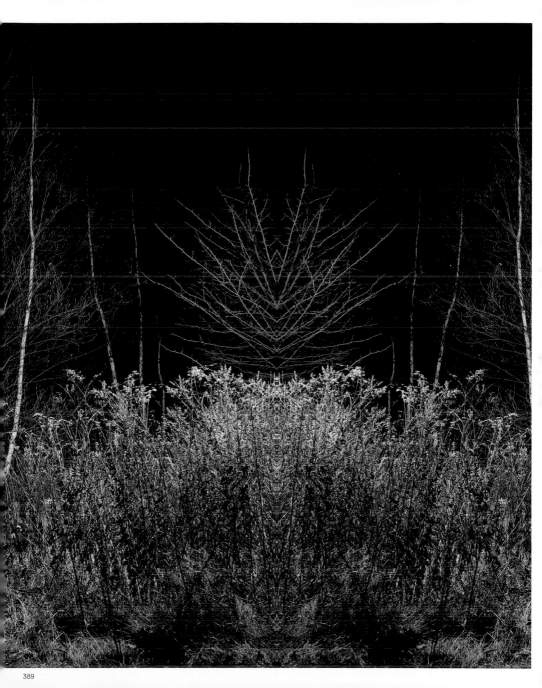

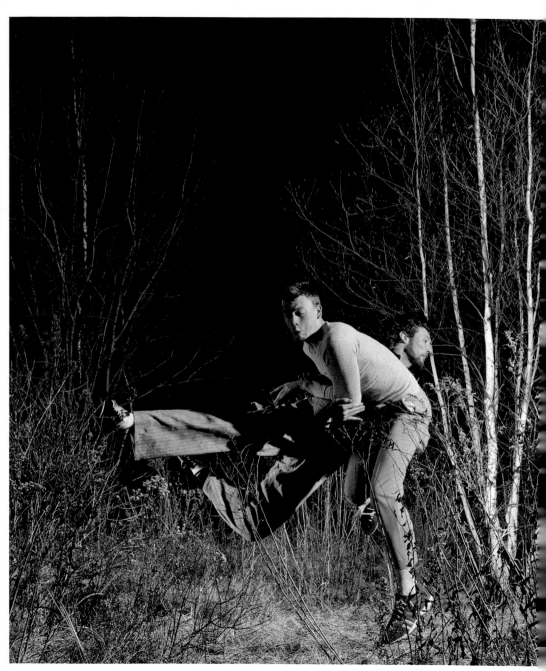

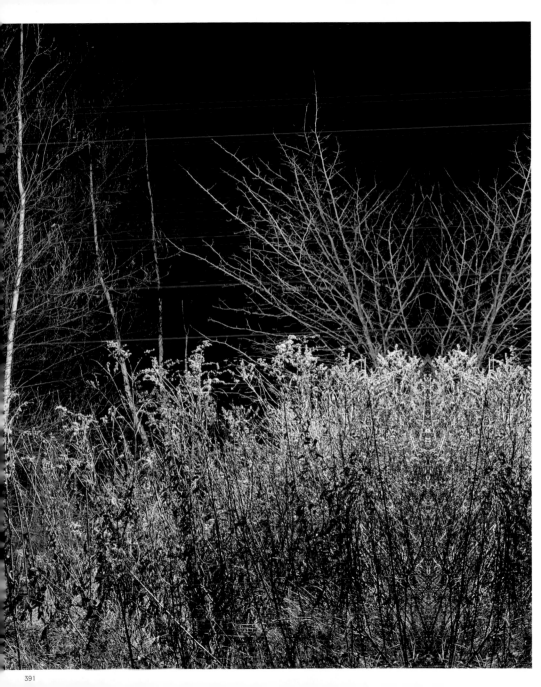

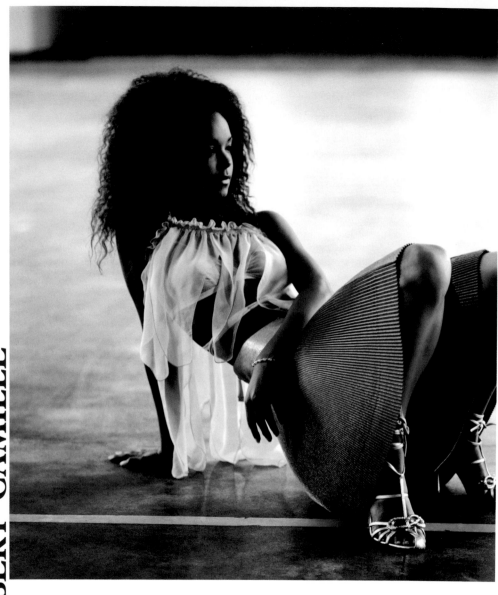

HUBERT CAMILLE

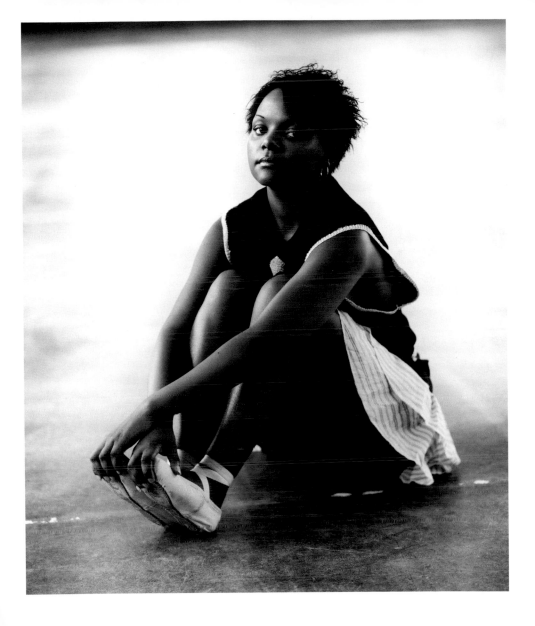

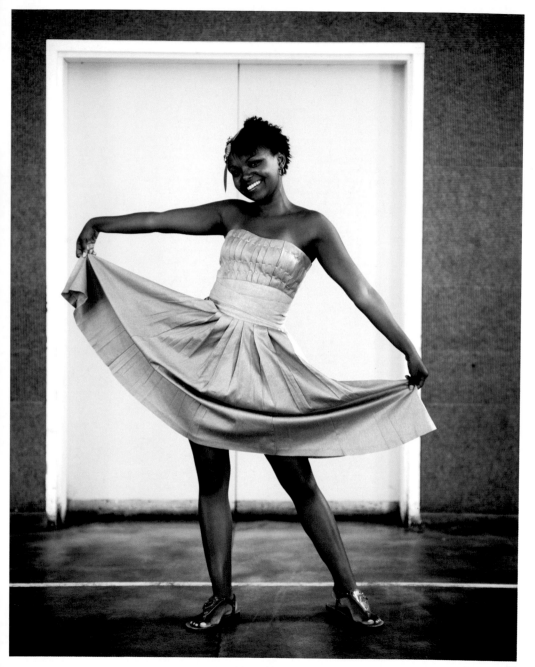

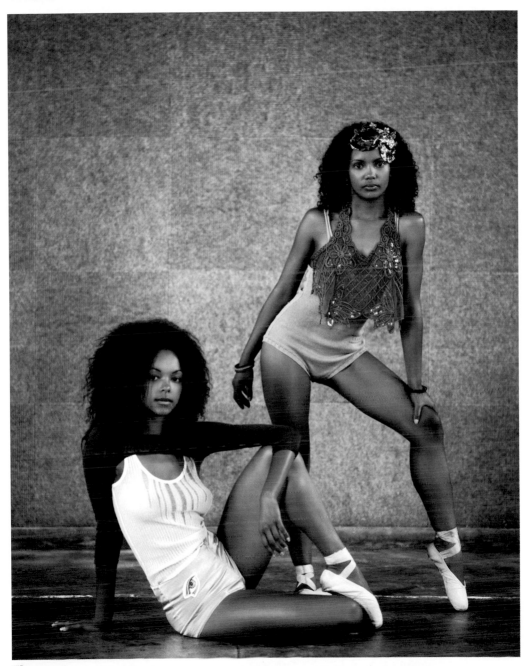

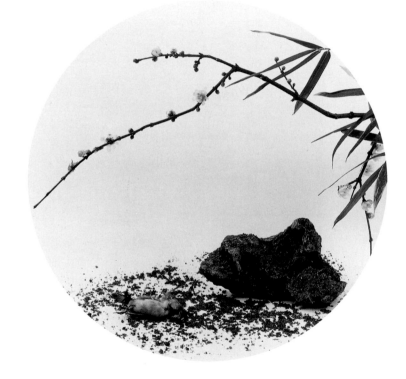

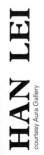

396

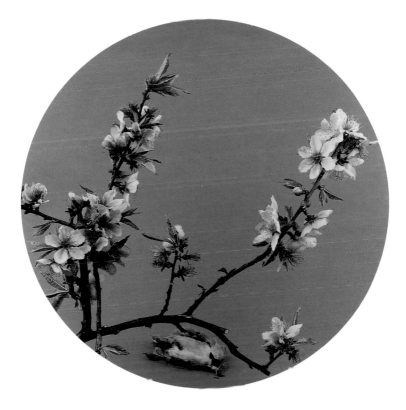

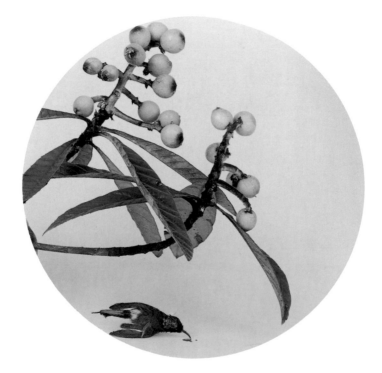

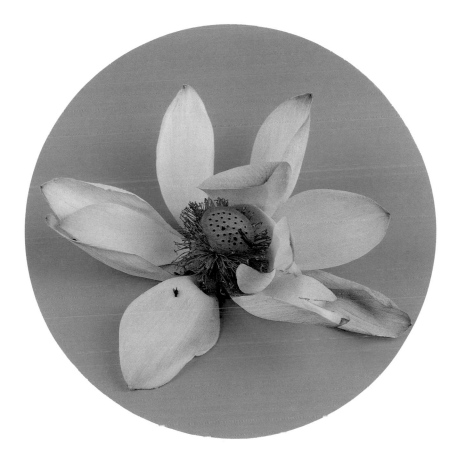

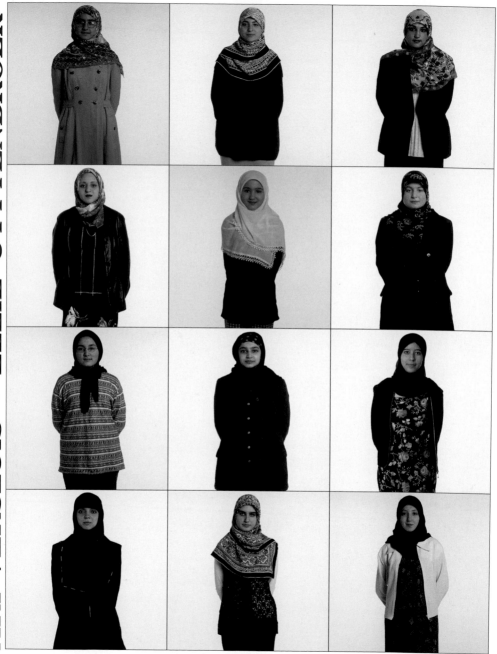

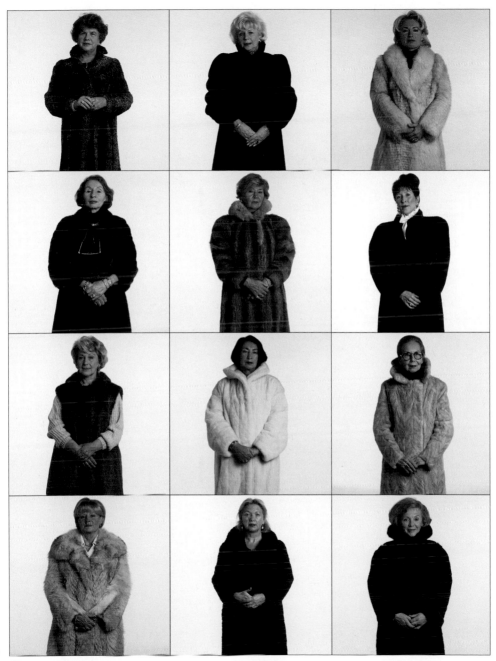

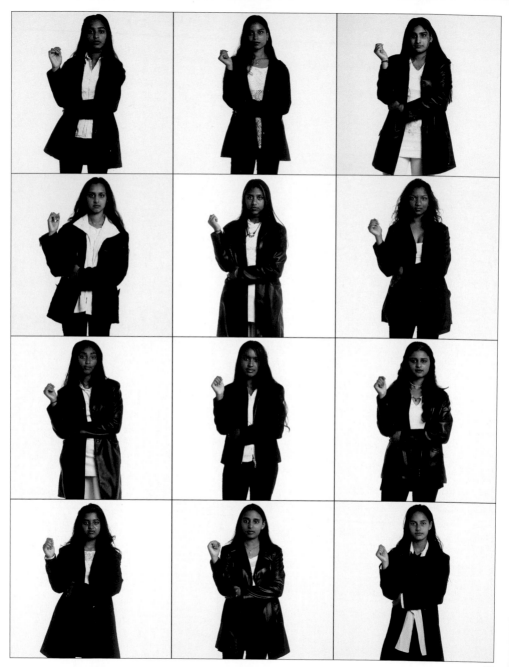

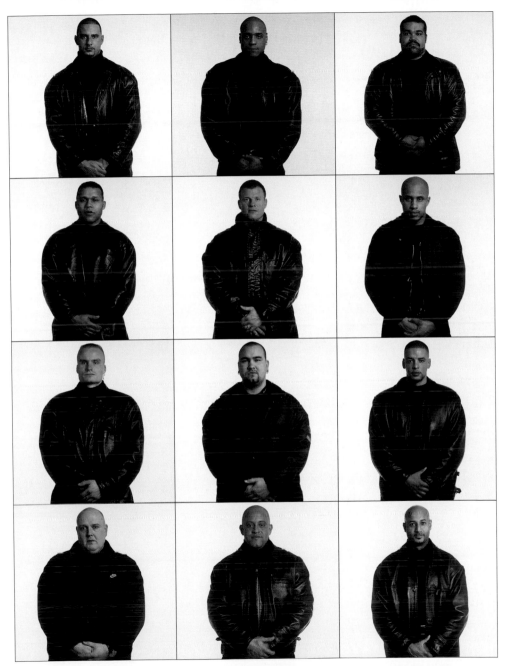

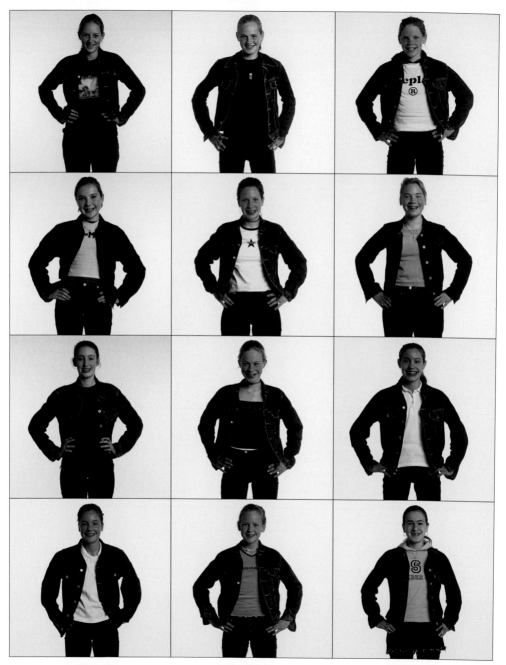

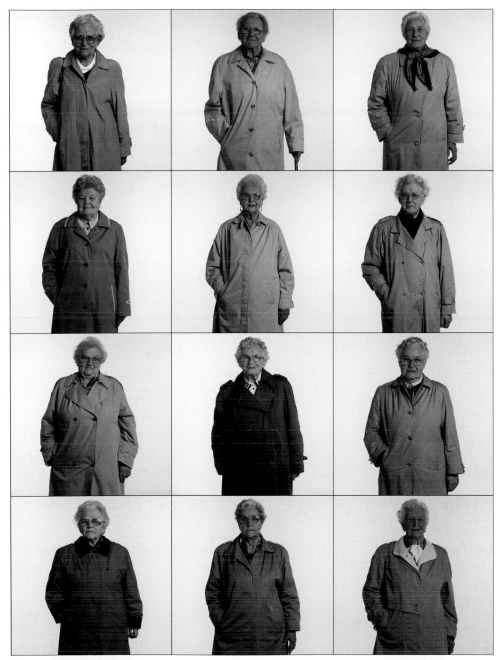

TANK

AVAILABLE IN GLORIOUS BLACK & WHITE

LITERATE

VOLUME 3 · ISSUE 7 · SEPTEMBER 2003 · COVER PHOTOGRAPH BY STEFANO GALUZZI

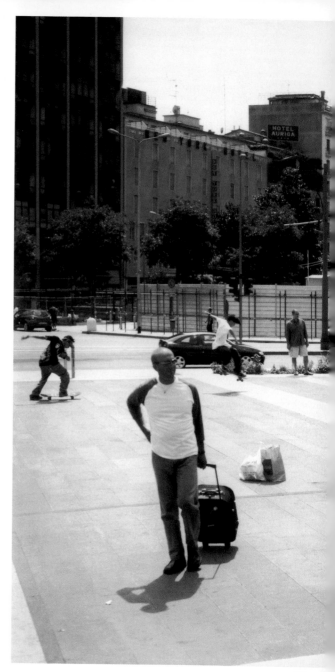

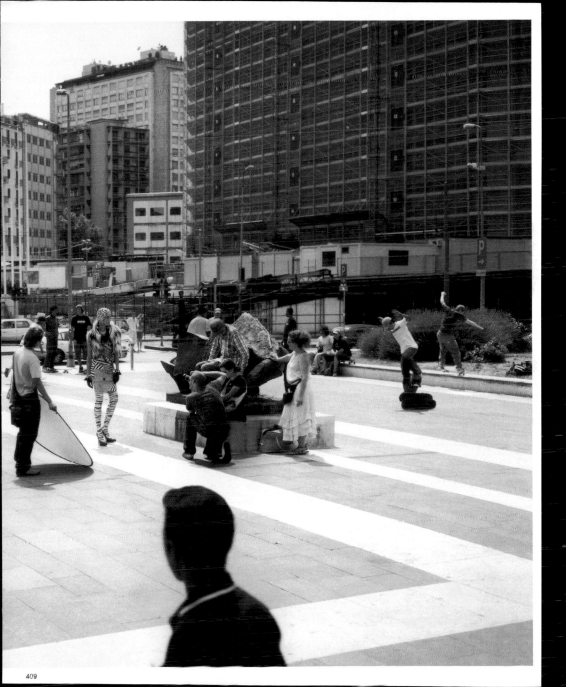

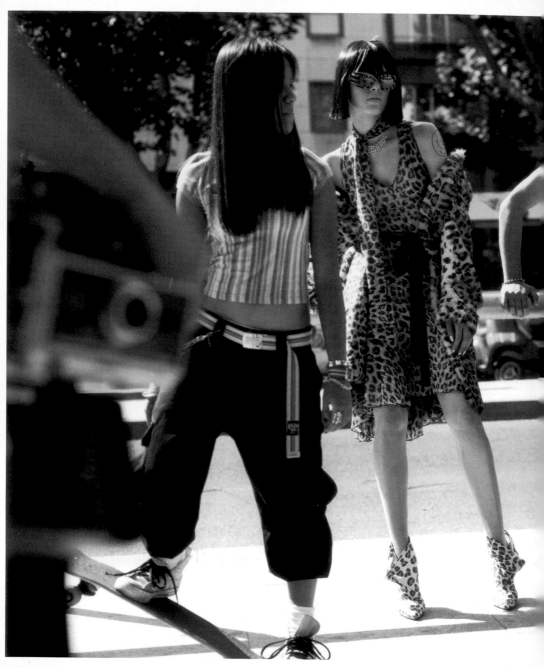

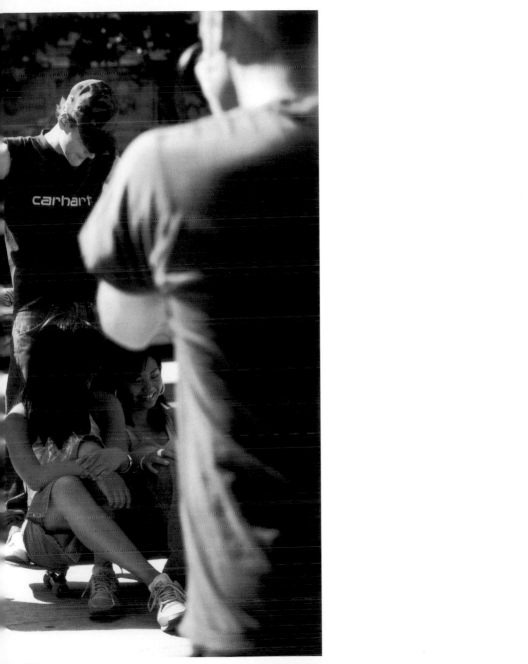

NEBOJSA SERIC-SHOBA

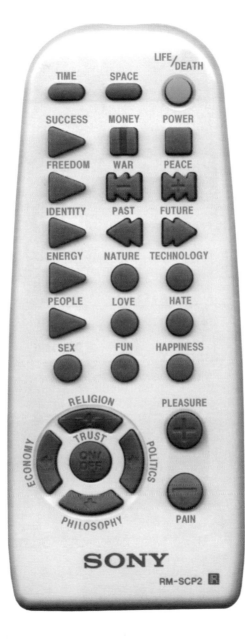

413

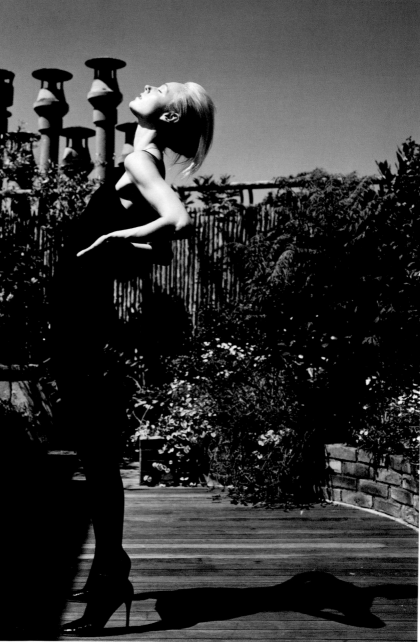

ERIC TRAORÉ

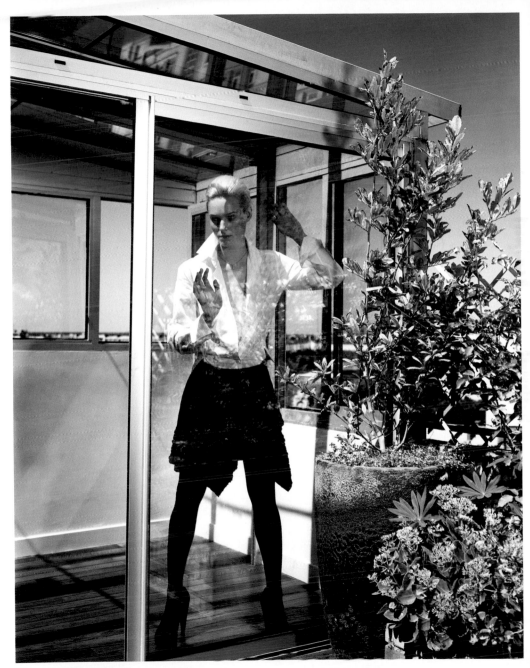

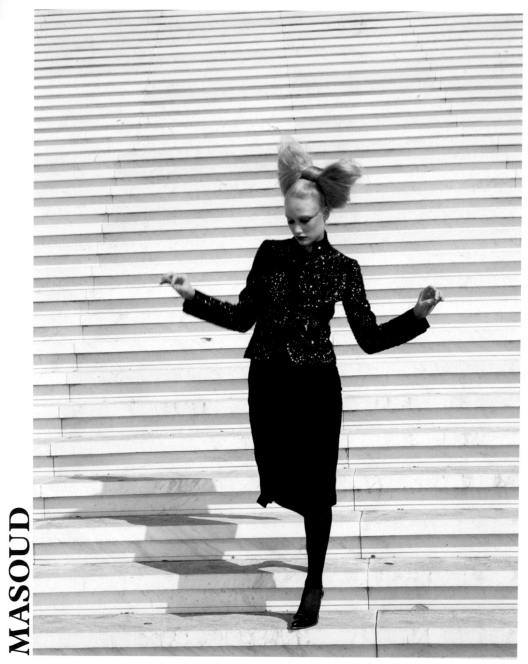

MASOUD

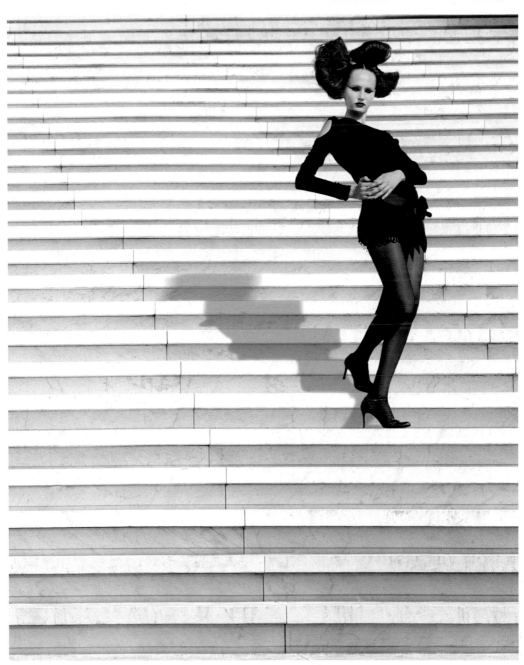

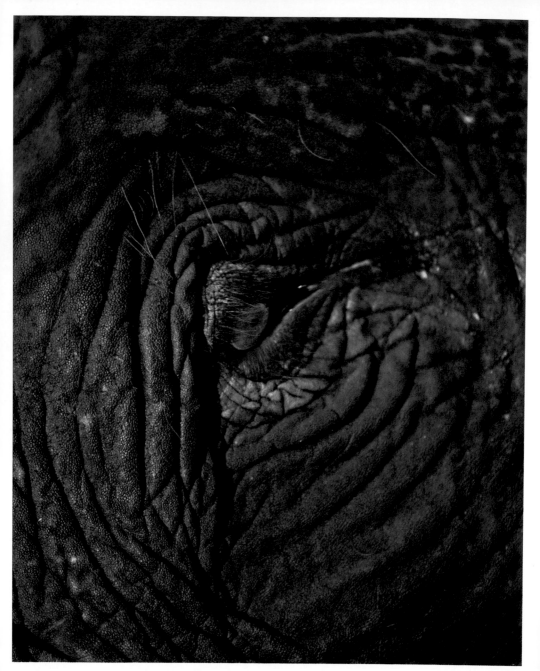

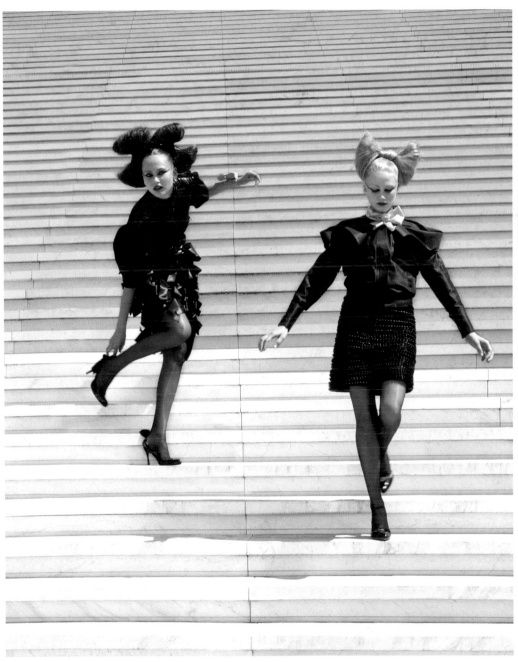

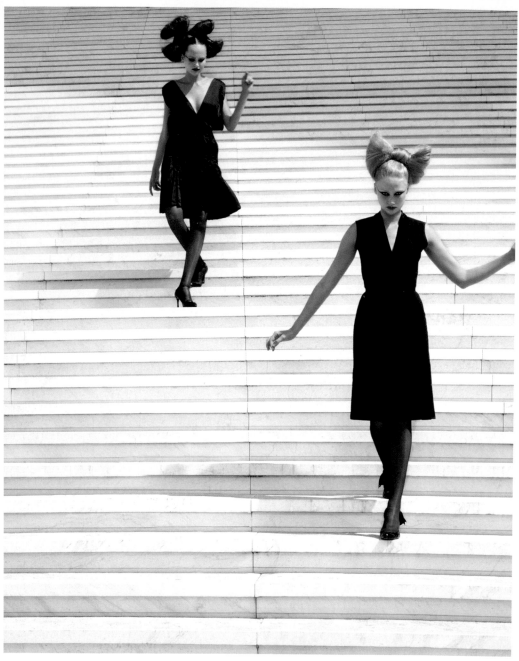

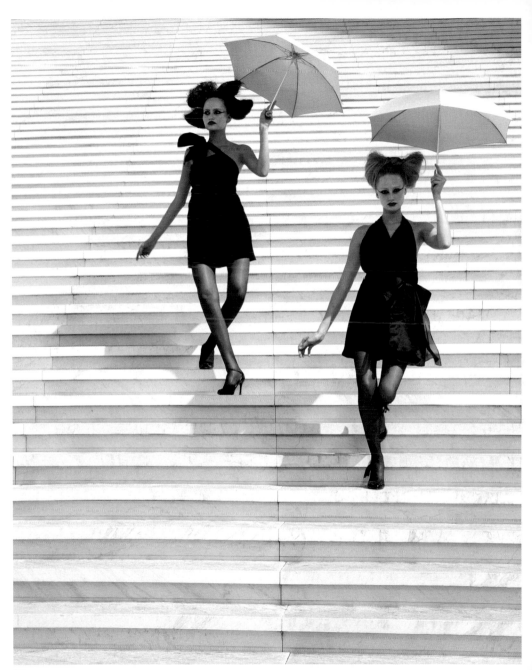

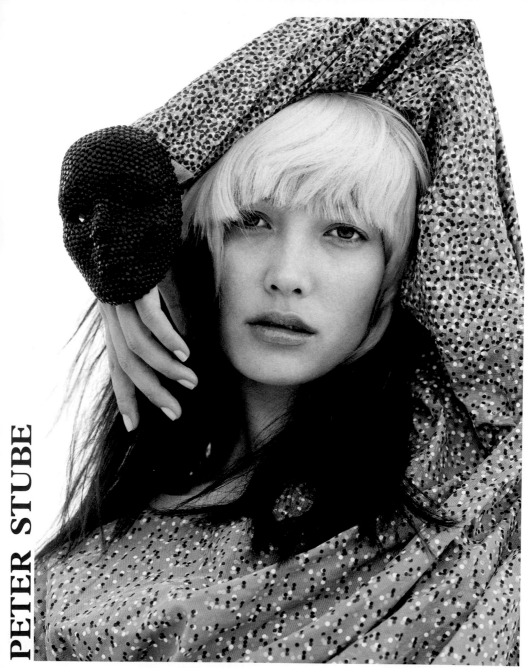

PETER STUBE

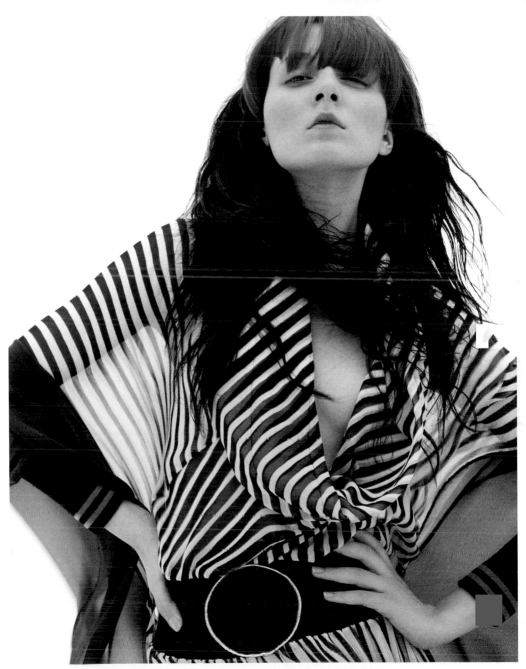

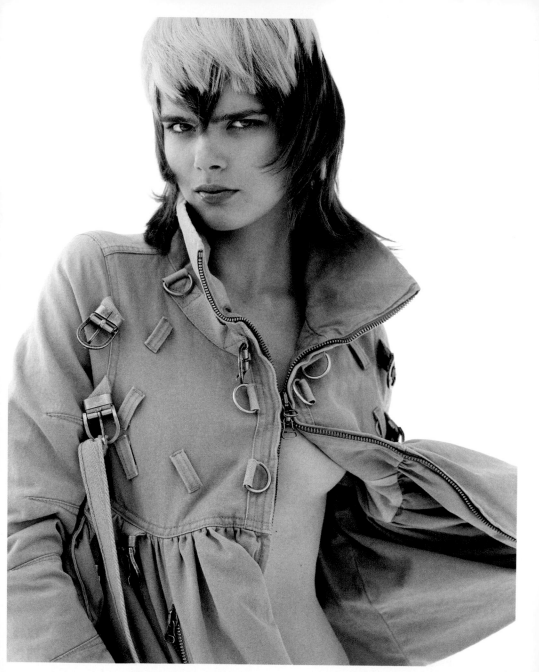

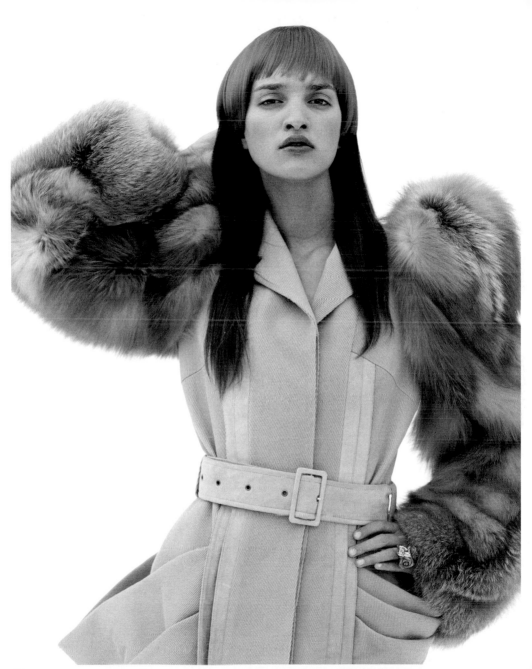

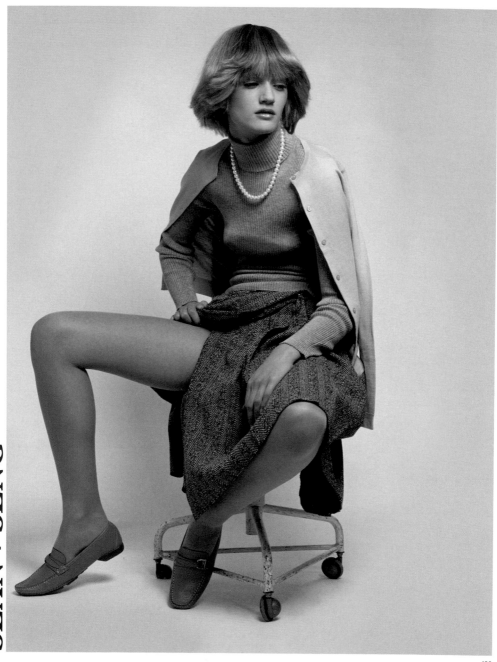

SEAN + SENG

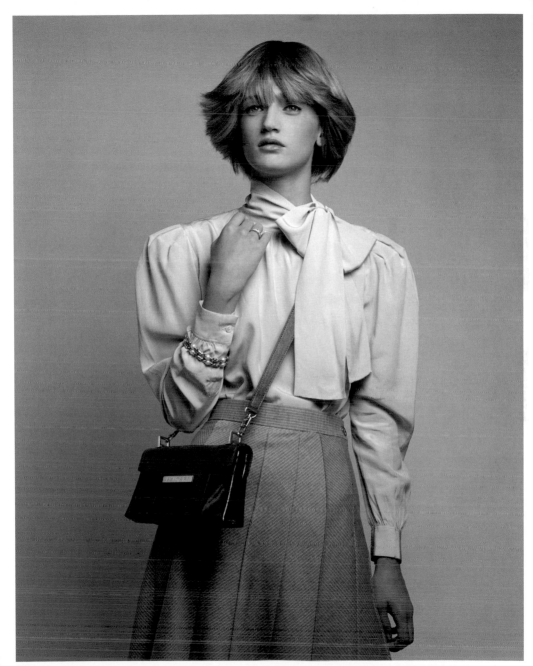

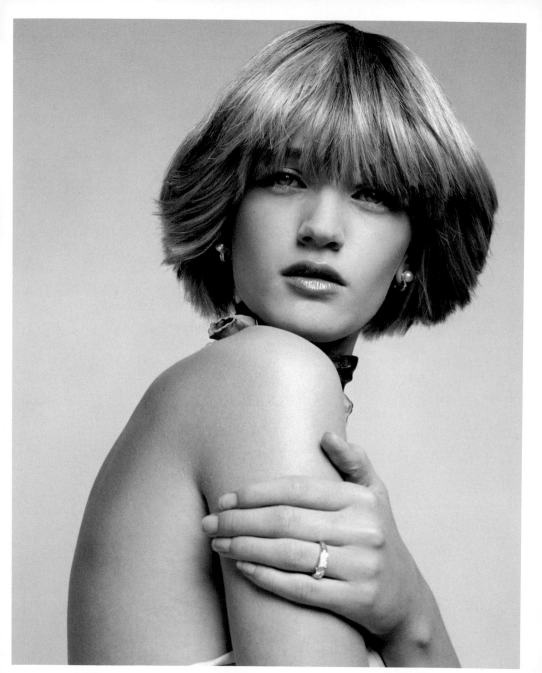

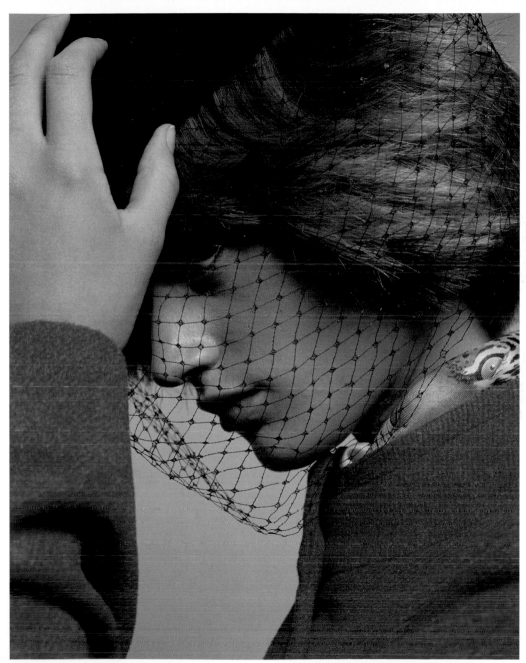

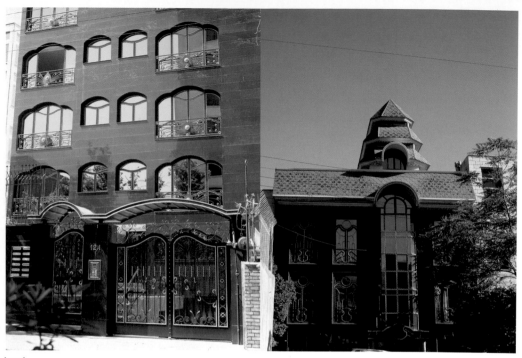

FARHAD MOSHIRI

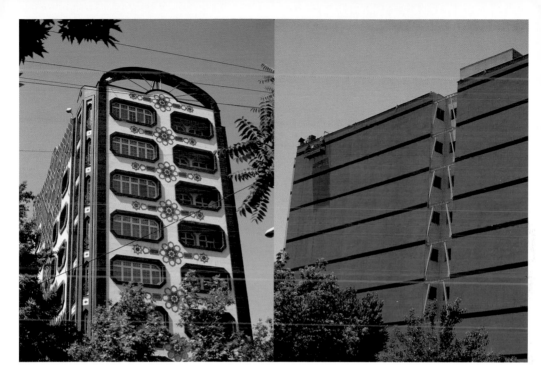

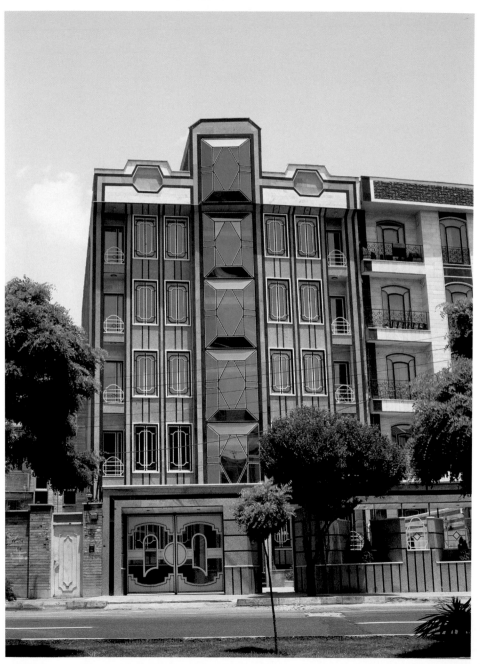

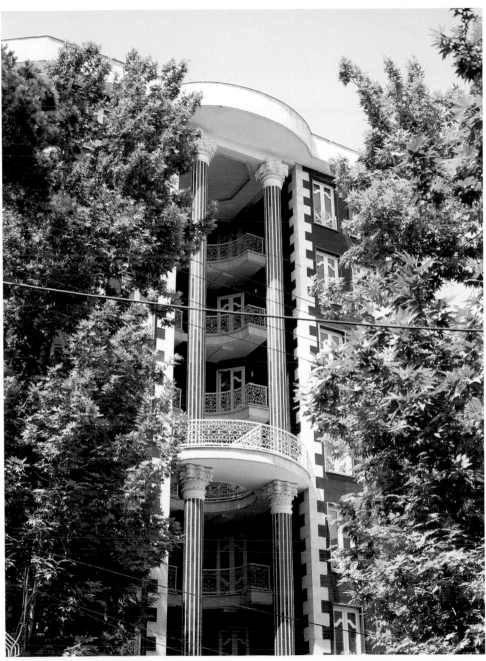

TONK

whYSL?

CORNUCOPIA

VOLUME 3 · ISSUE 8 · DECEMBER 2003 · COVER PHOTOGRAPH BY STEFANO GALUZZI

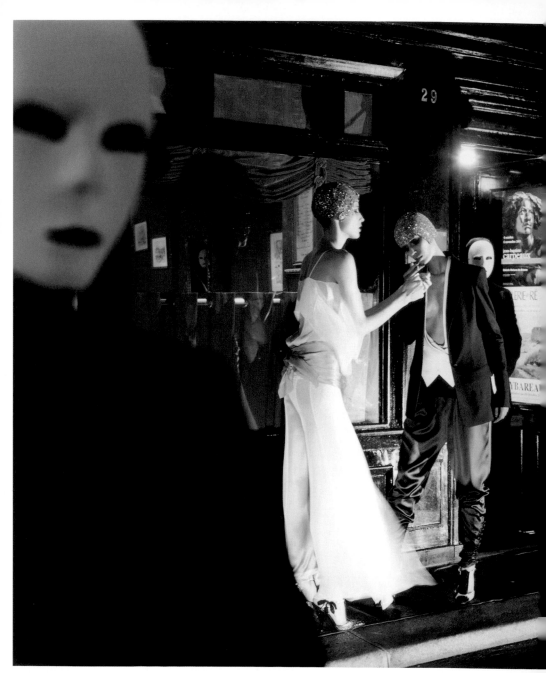

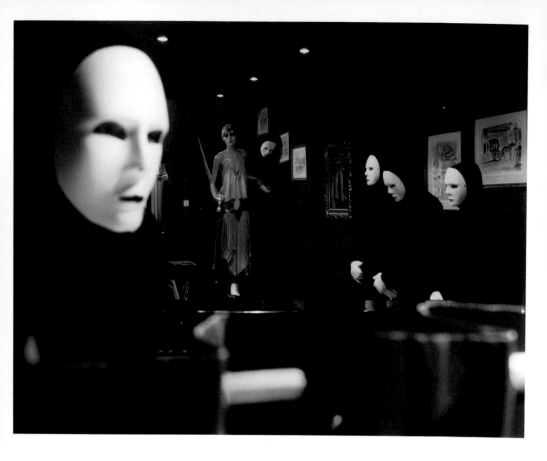

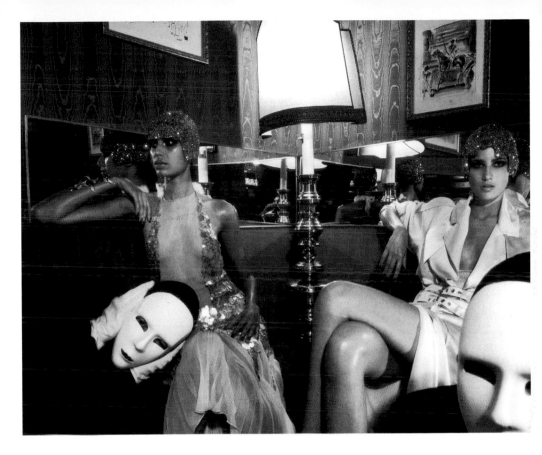

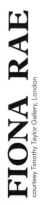

FIONA RAE

courtesy Timothy Taylor Gallery, London

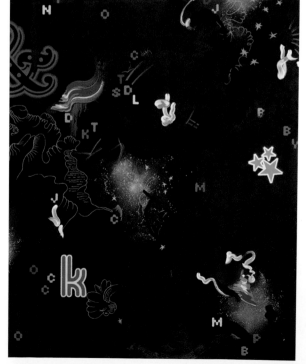

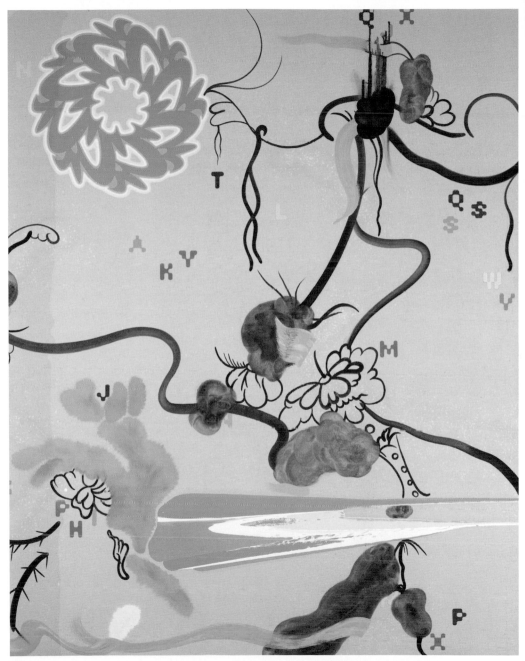

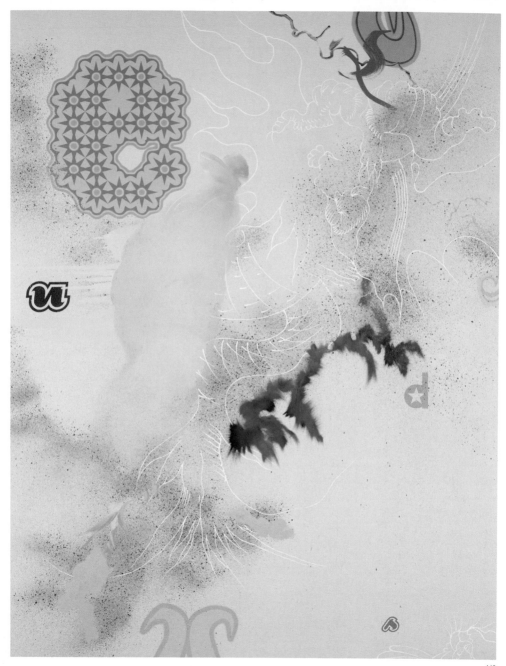

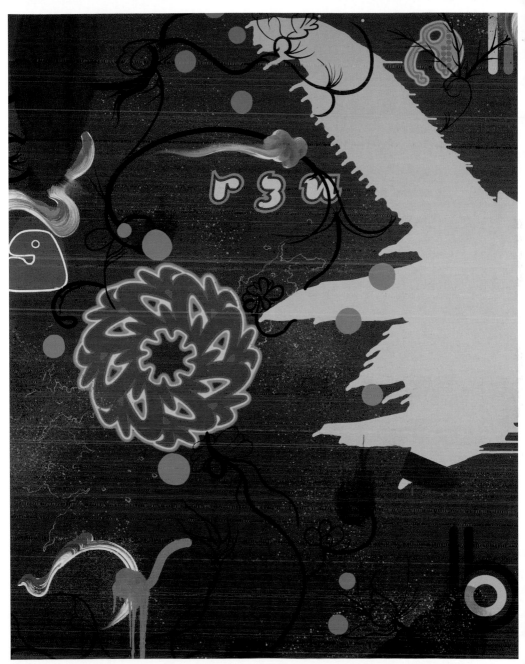

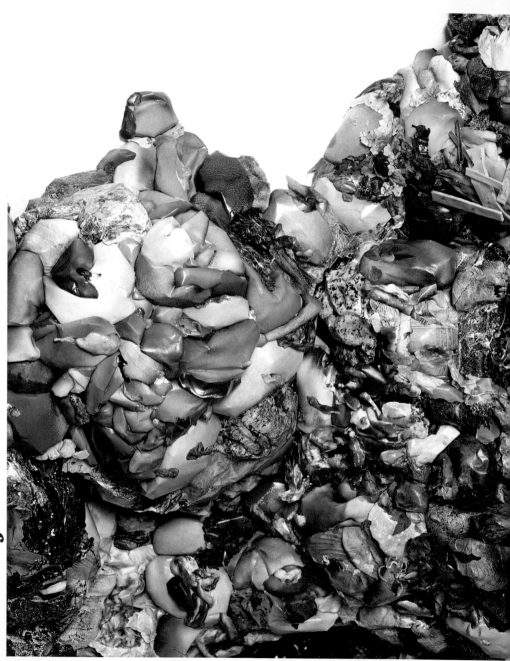

CHRIS JONES

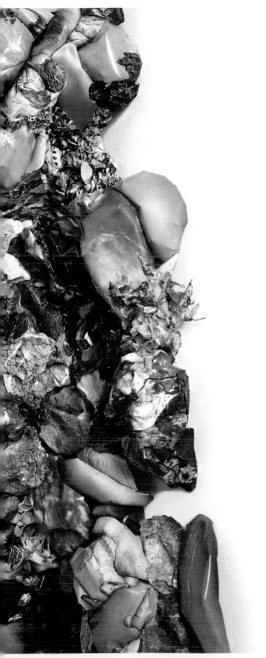

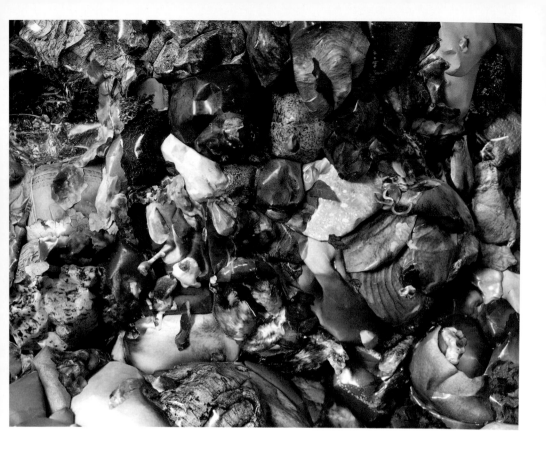

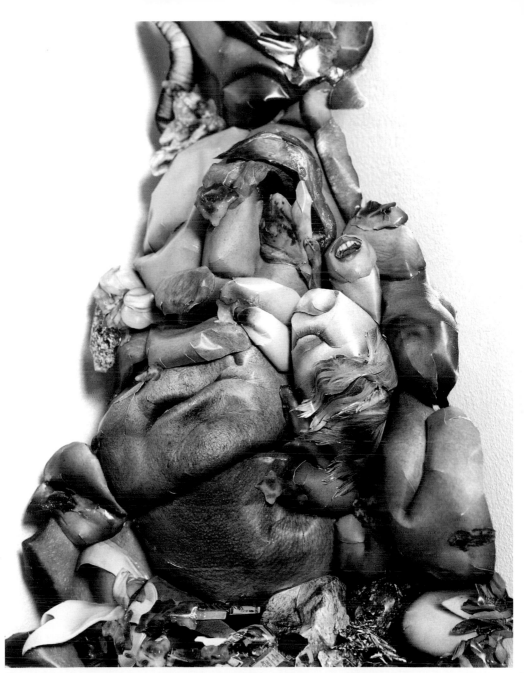

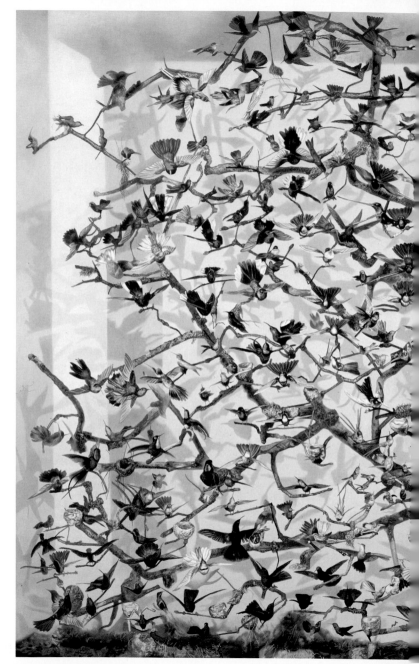

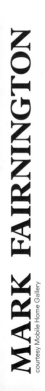

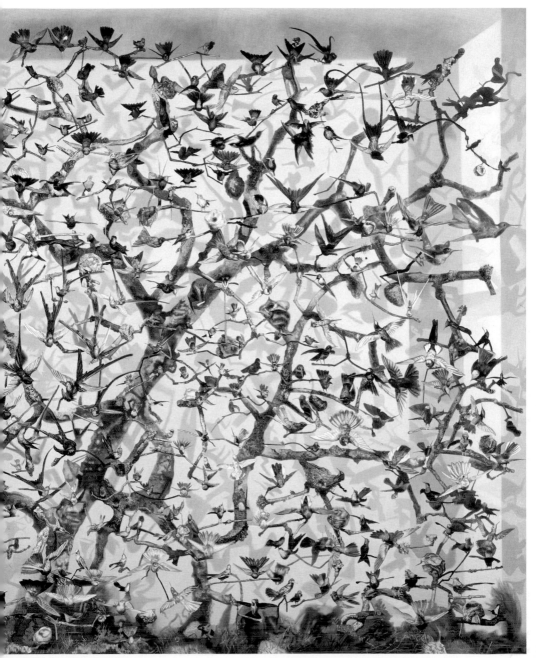

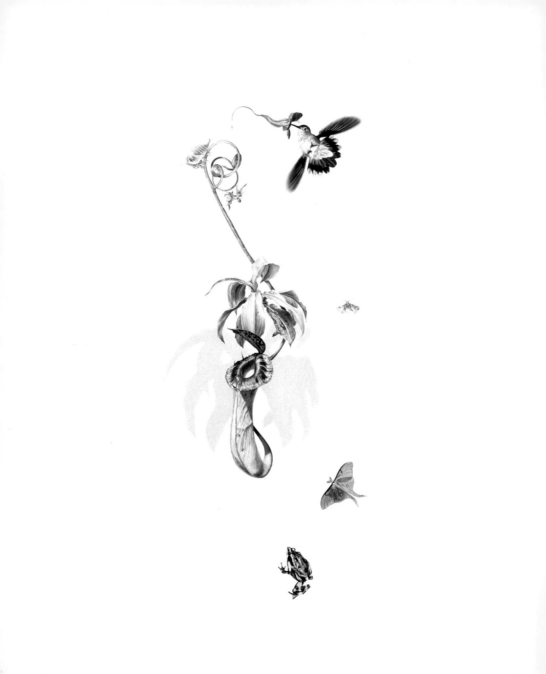

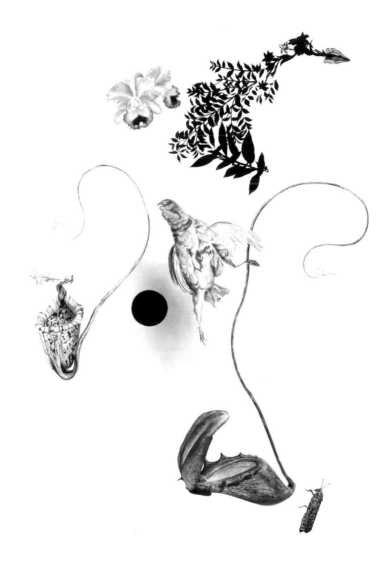

CAMILLE KERBELLEC

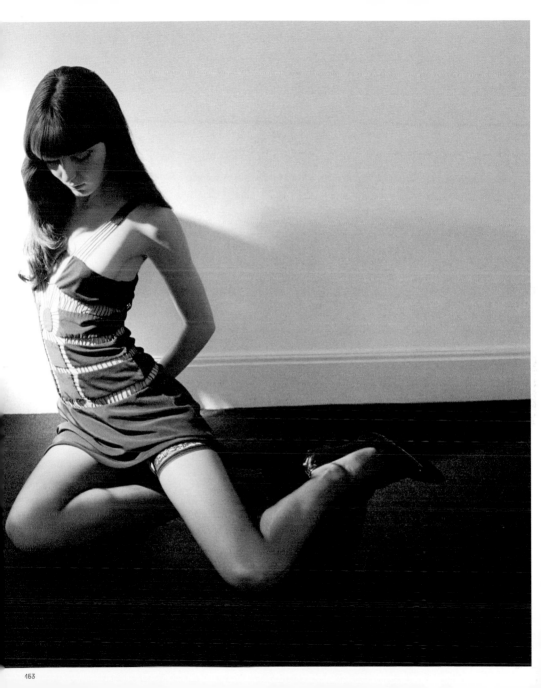

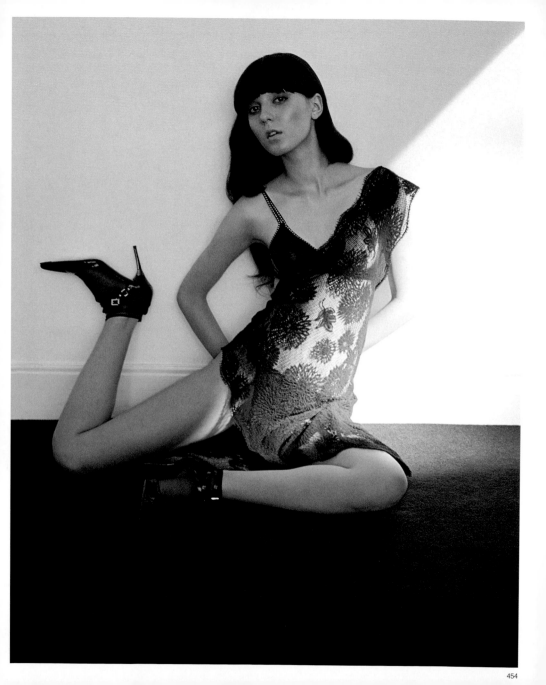

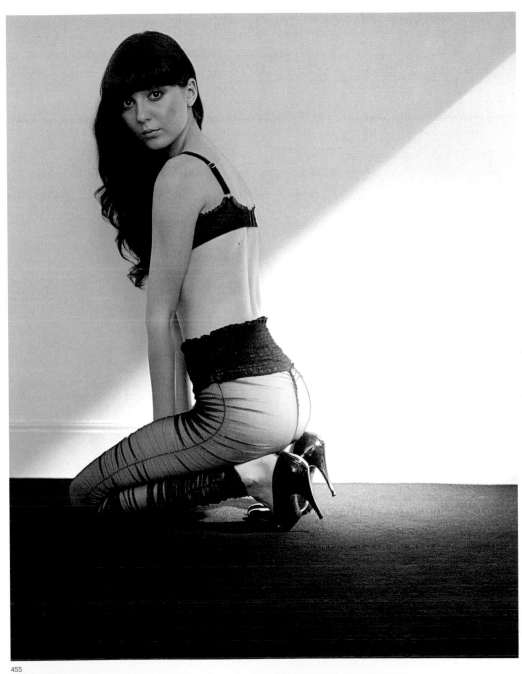

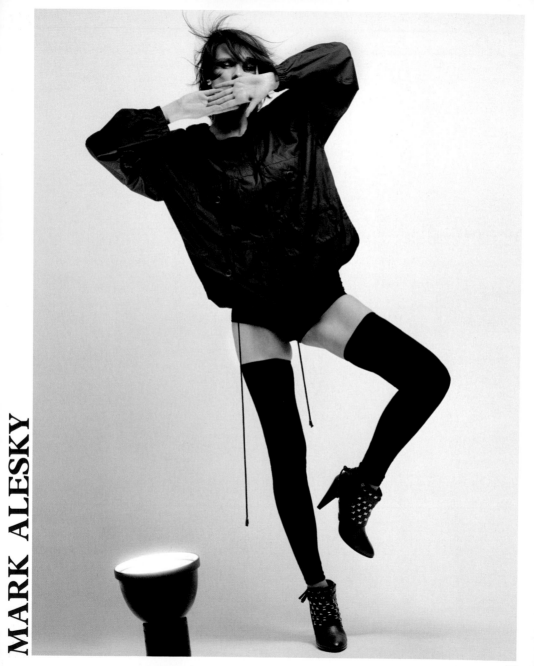

MARK ALESKY

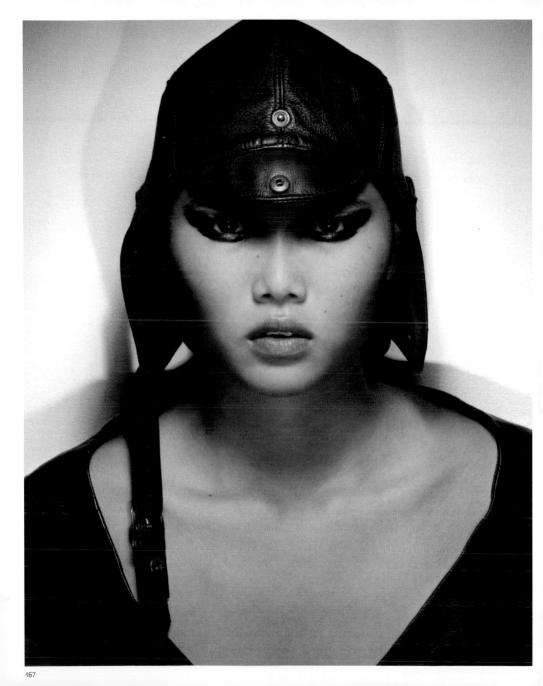

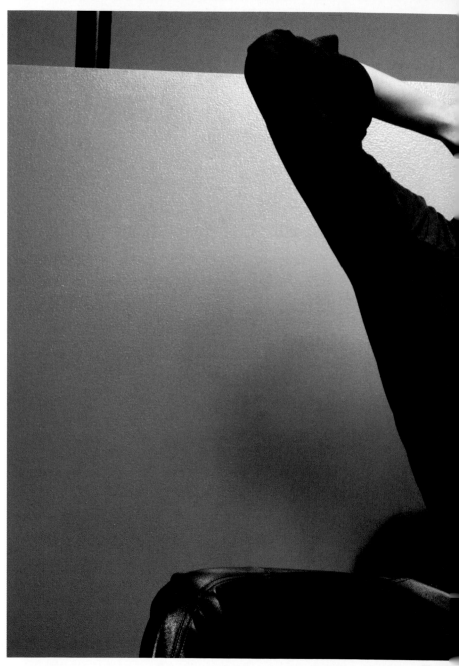

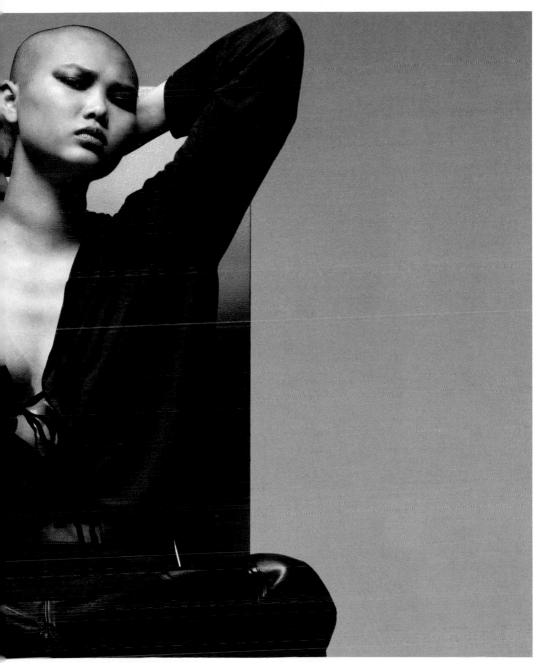

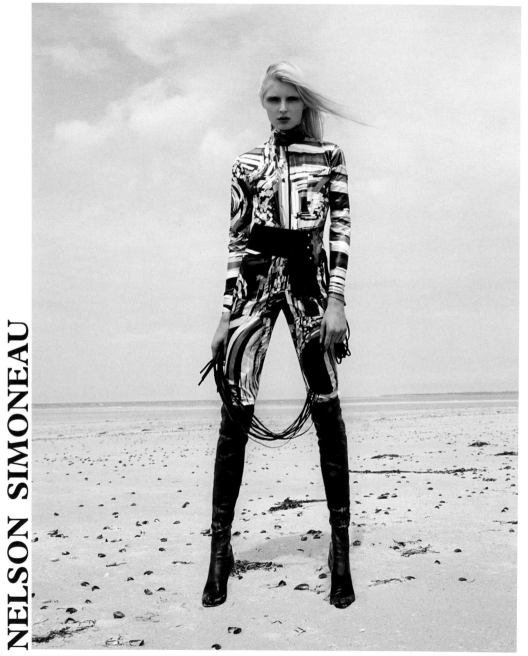

NELSON SIMONEAU

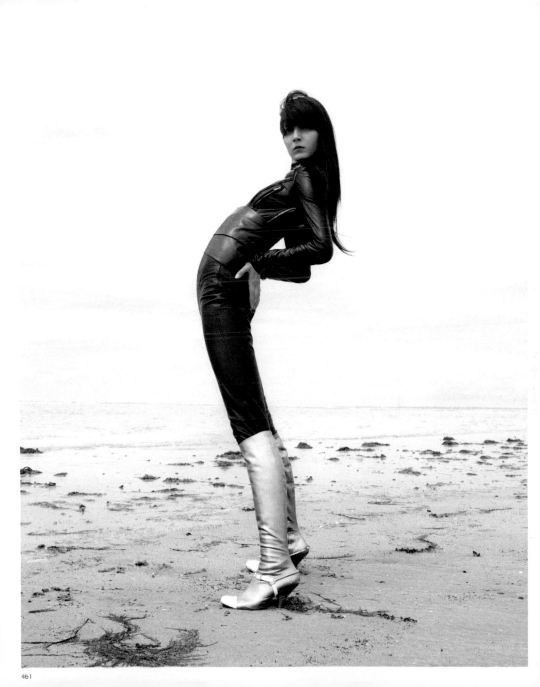

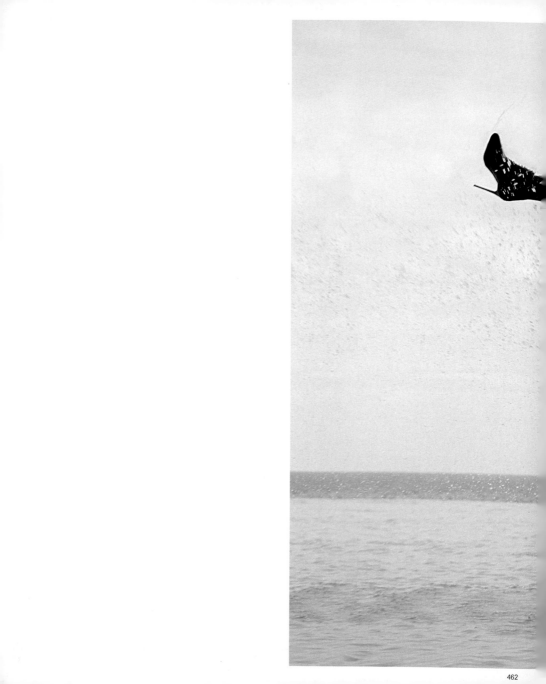

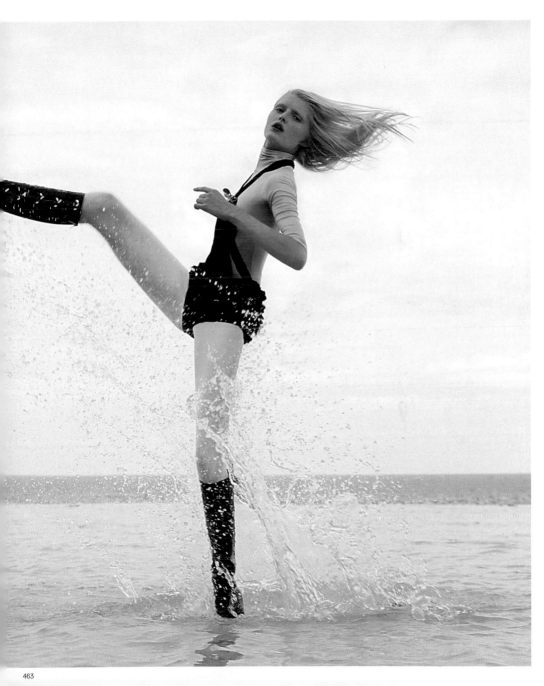

VOLUME 3 · ISSUE 9 · £10

TANK

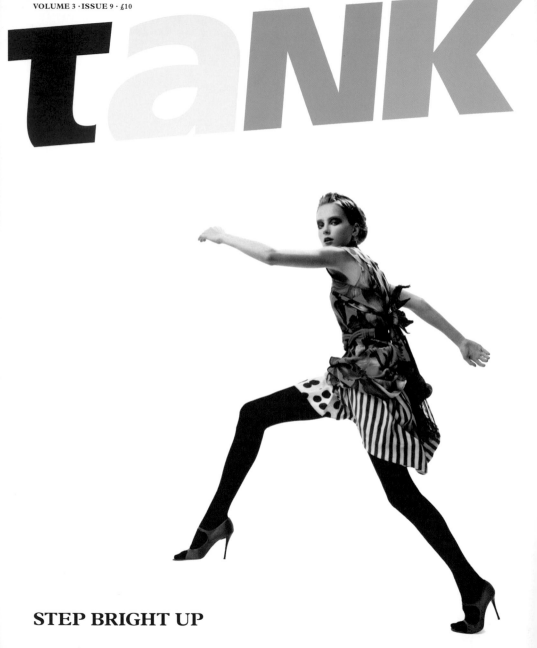

STEP BRIGHT UP

SPRING LOADED

VOLUME 3 · ISSUE 9 · MARCH 2004 · COVER PHOTOGRAPH BY MARIANO VIVANCO

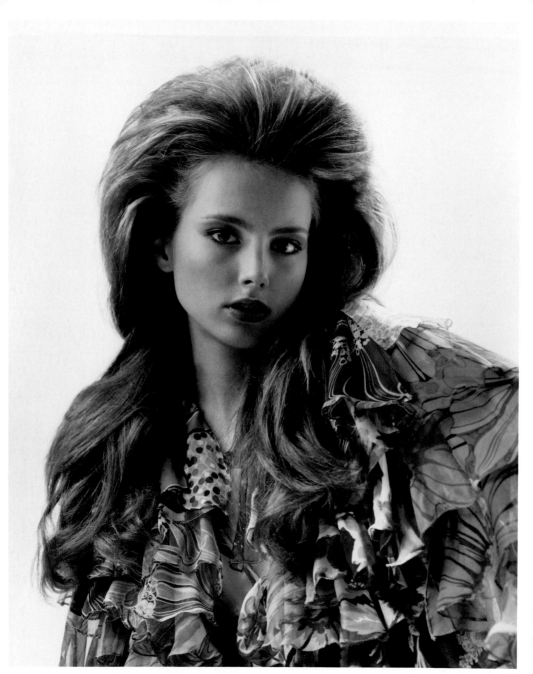

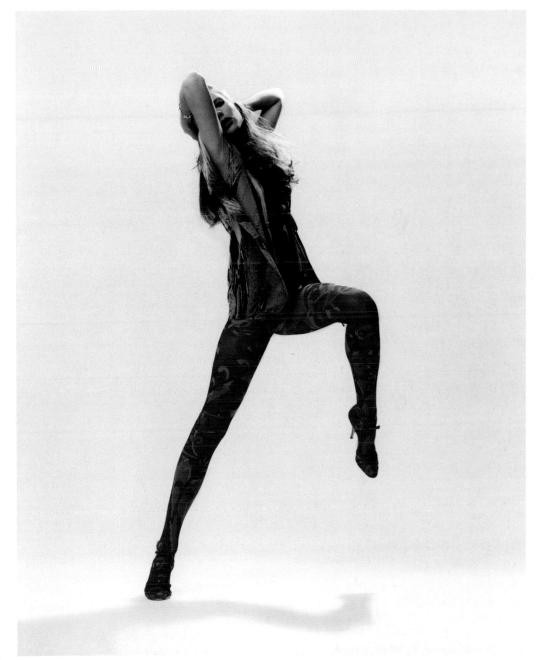

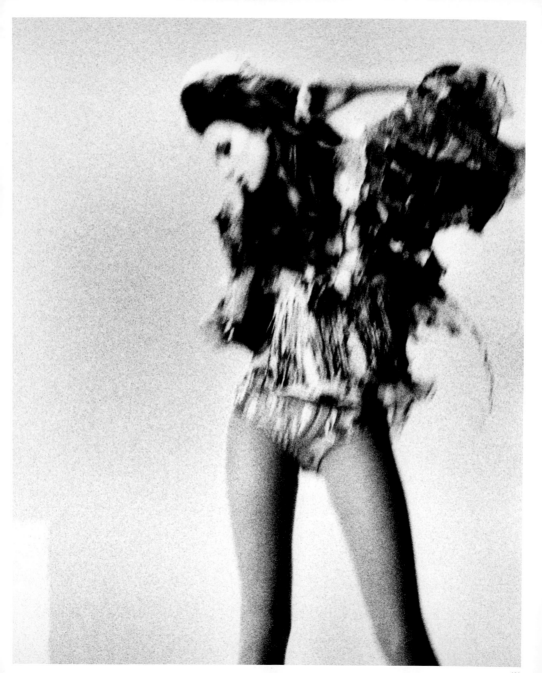

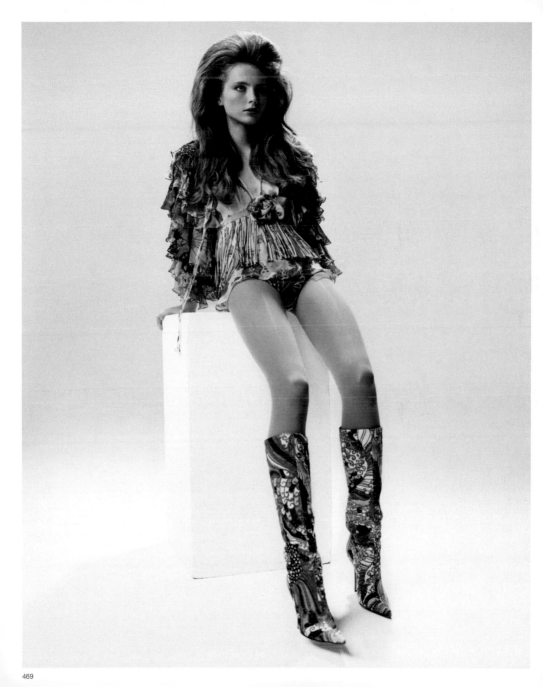

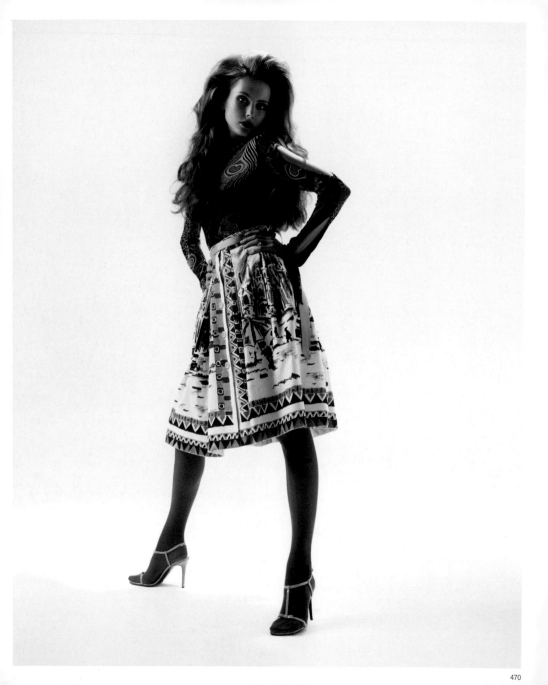

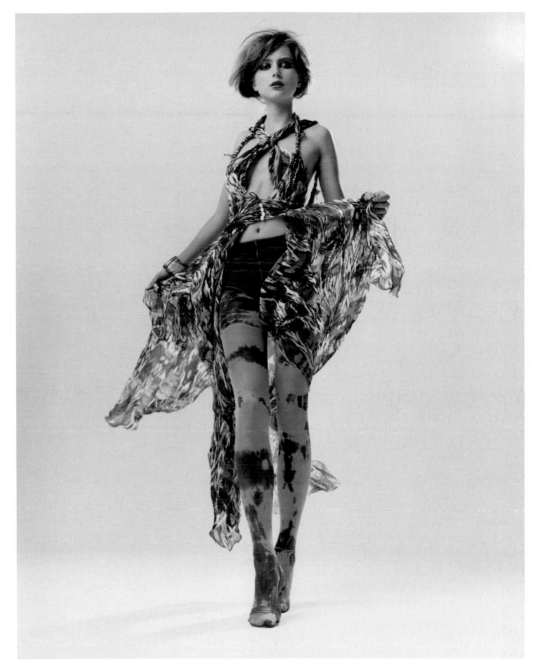

THIERRY VAN BIESEN

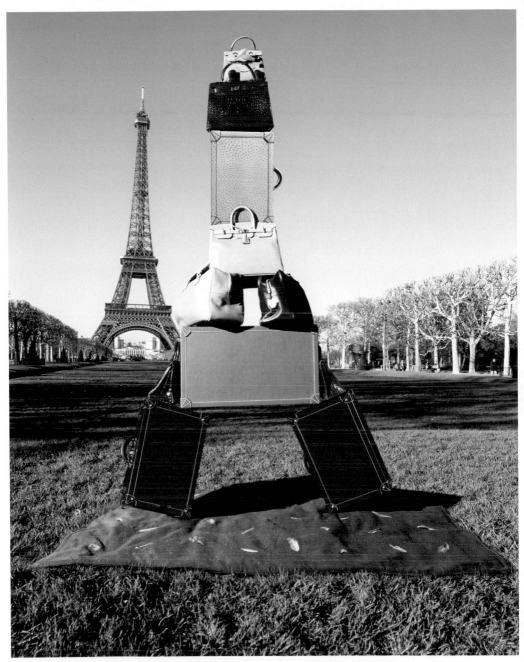

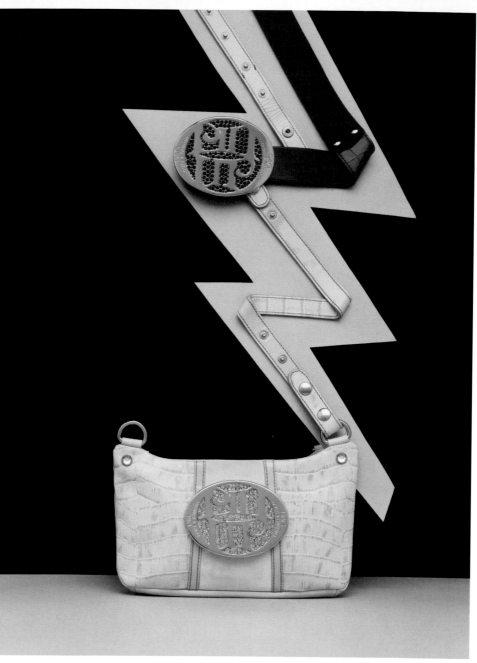

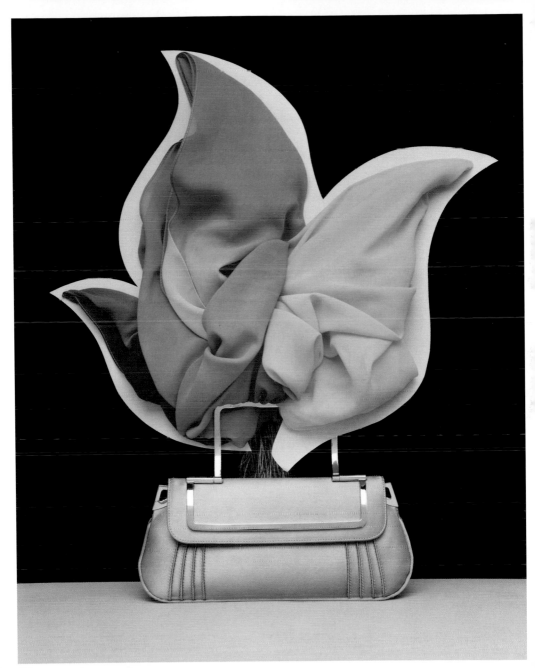

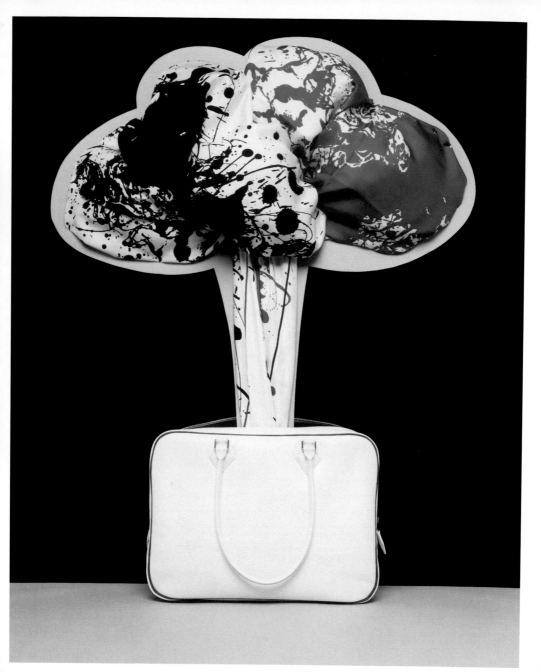

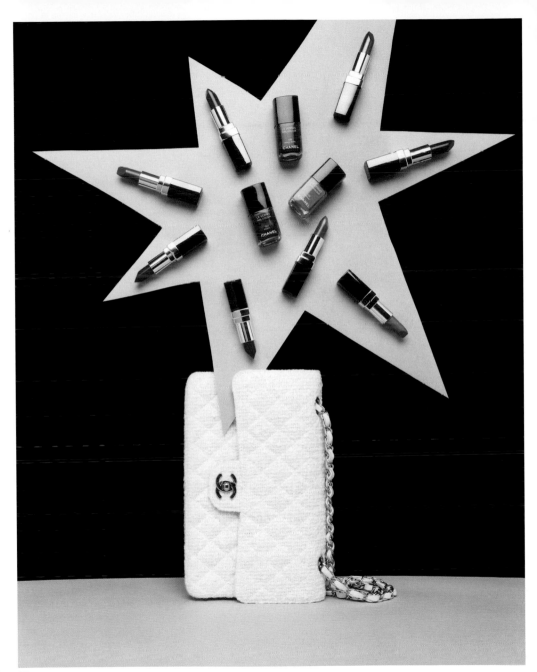

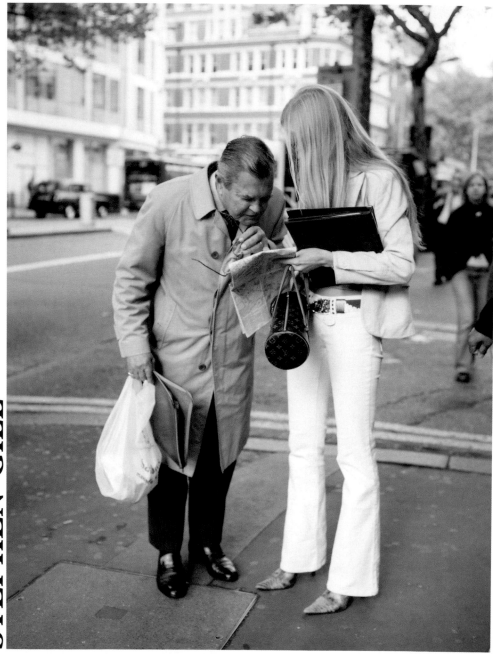

STEPHEN GILL

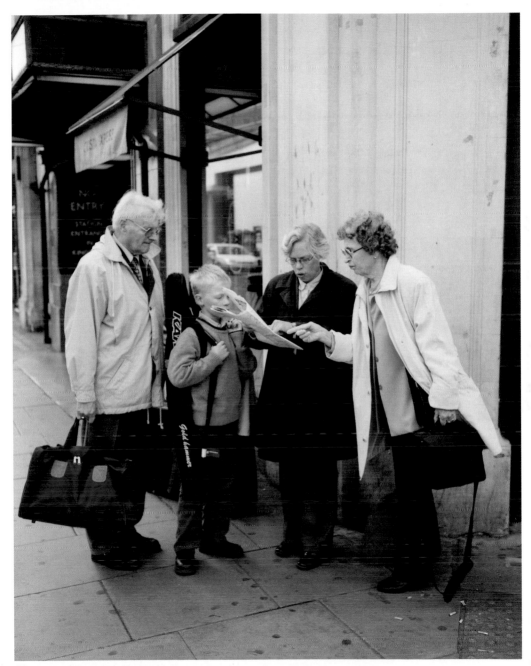

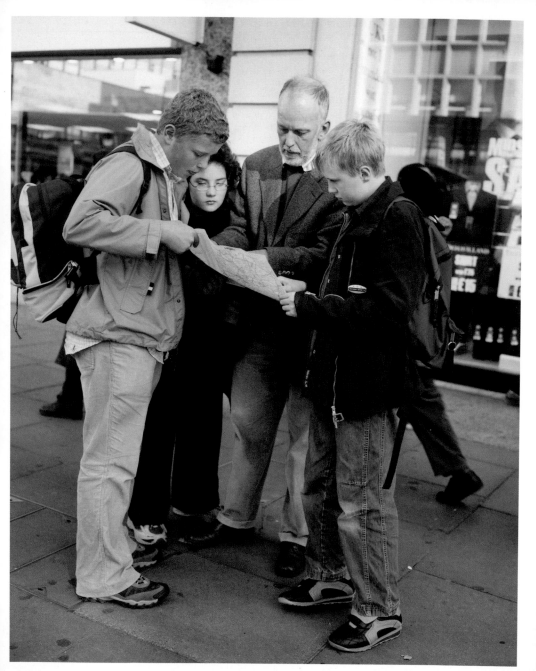

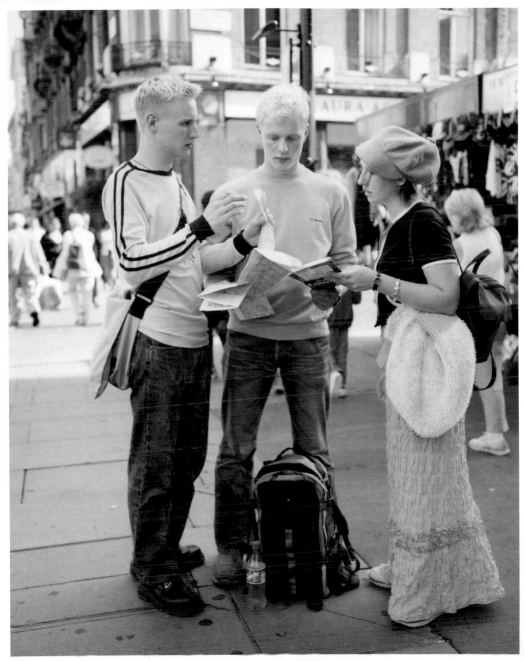

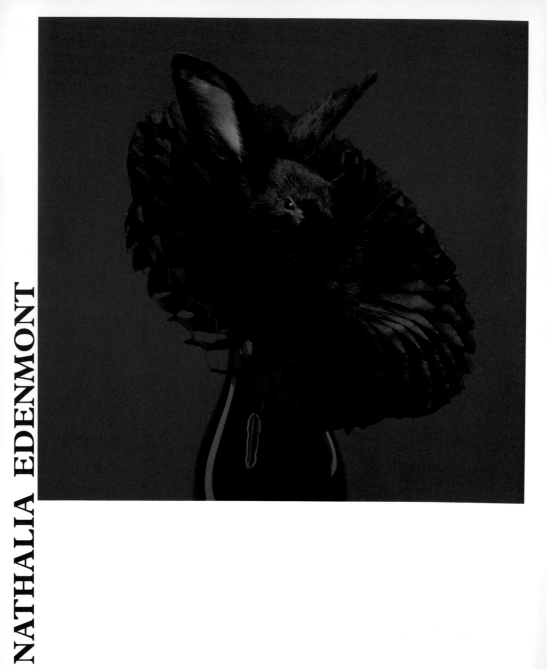

NATHALIA EDENMONT

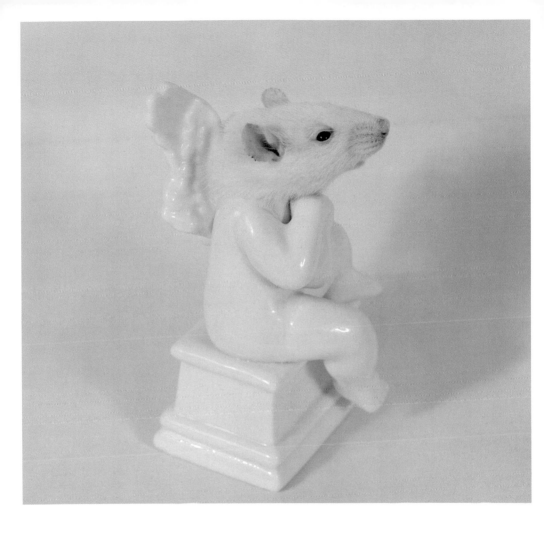

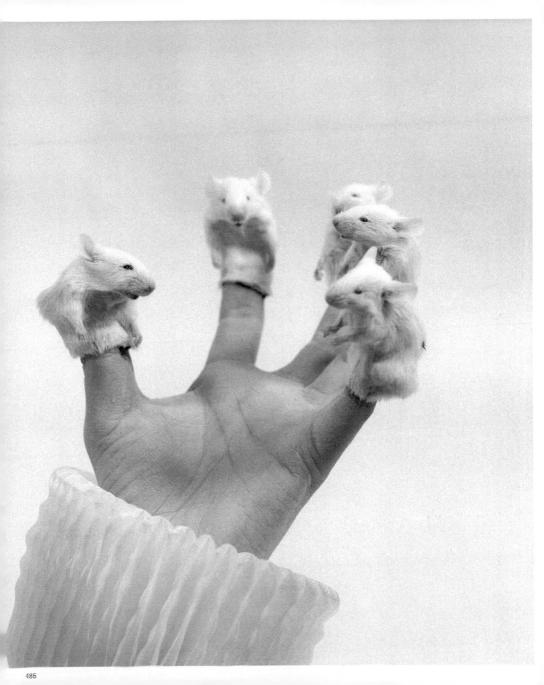

RICHARD BILLINGHAM

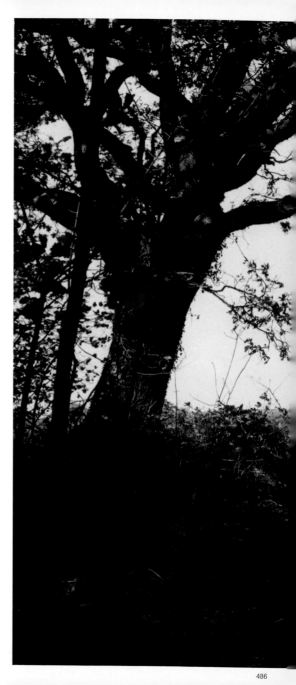

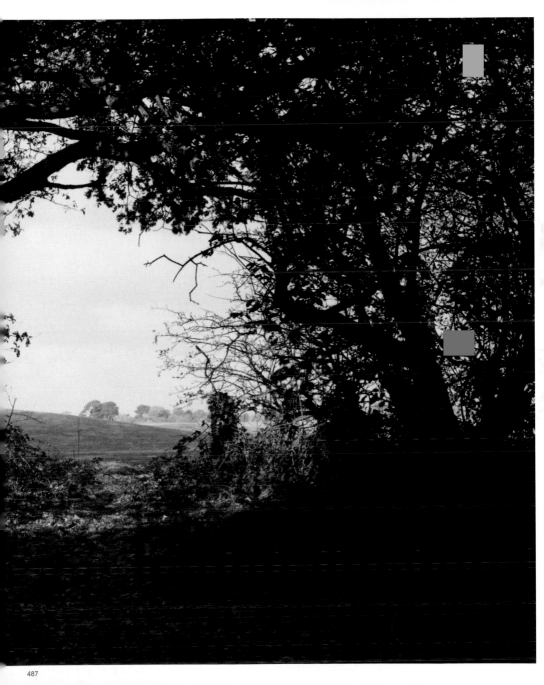

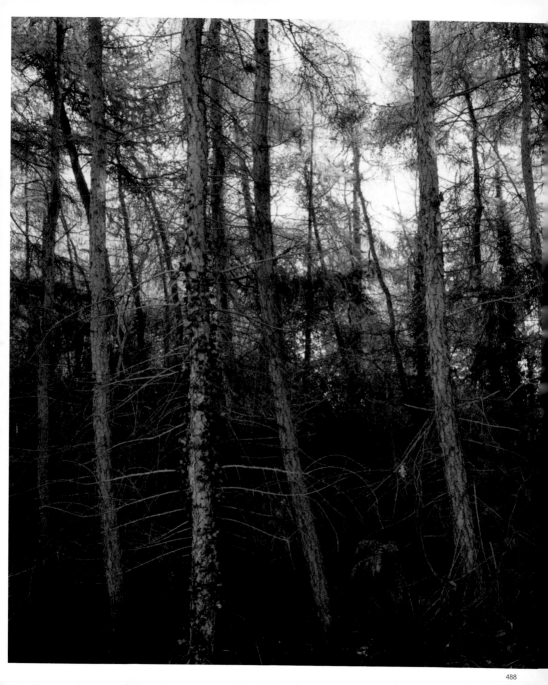

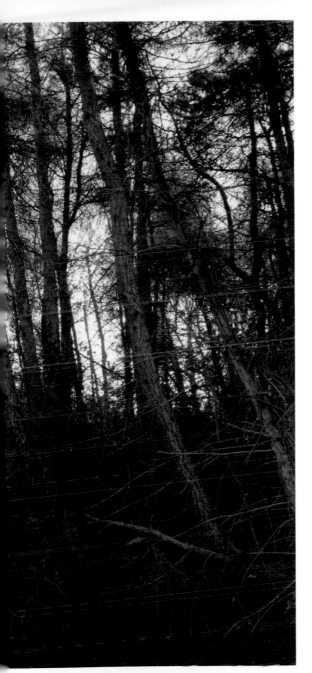

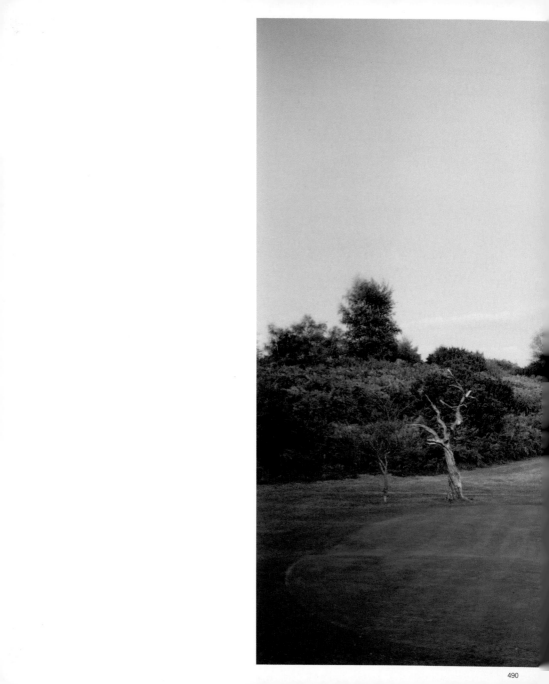

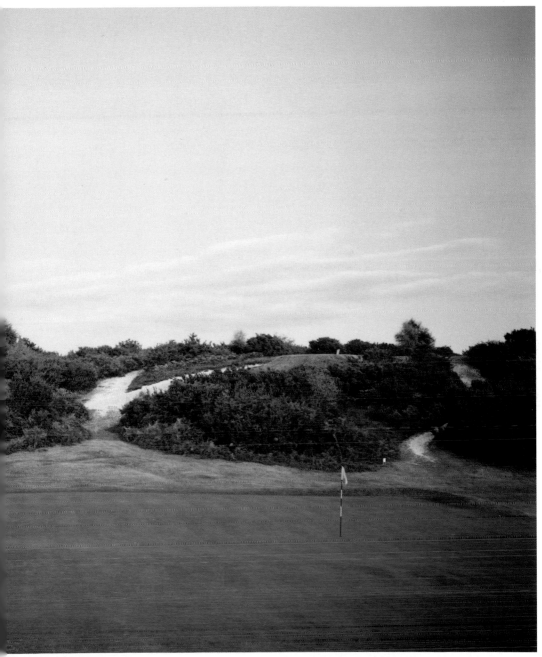

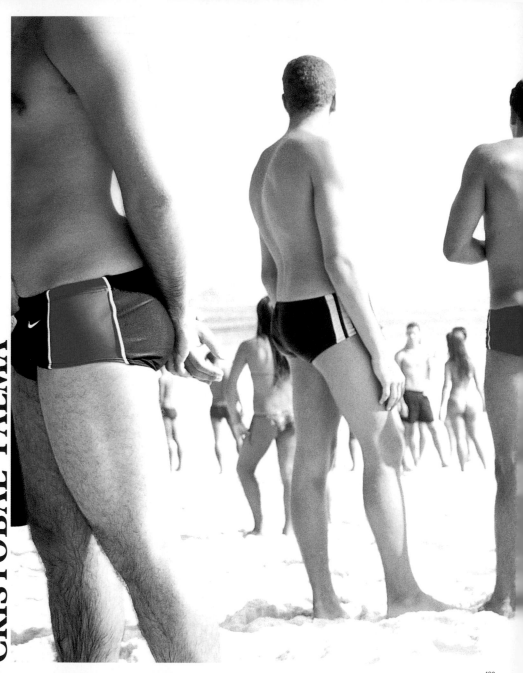

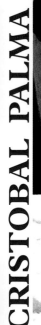

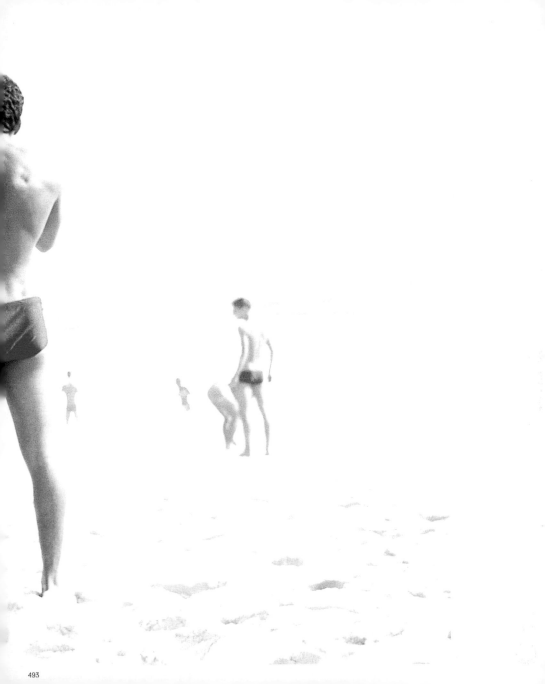

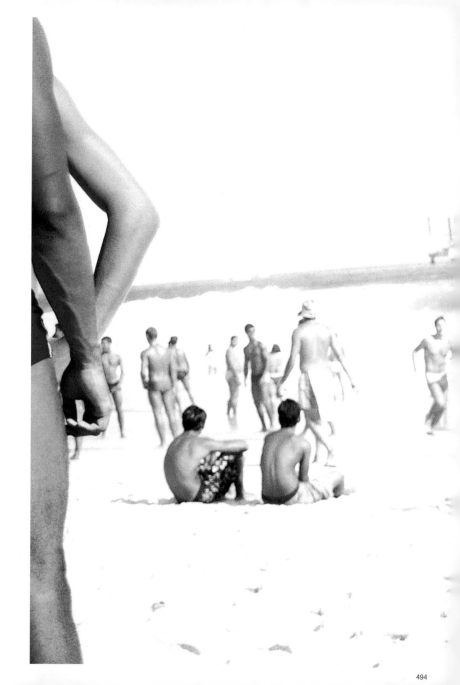

494

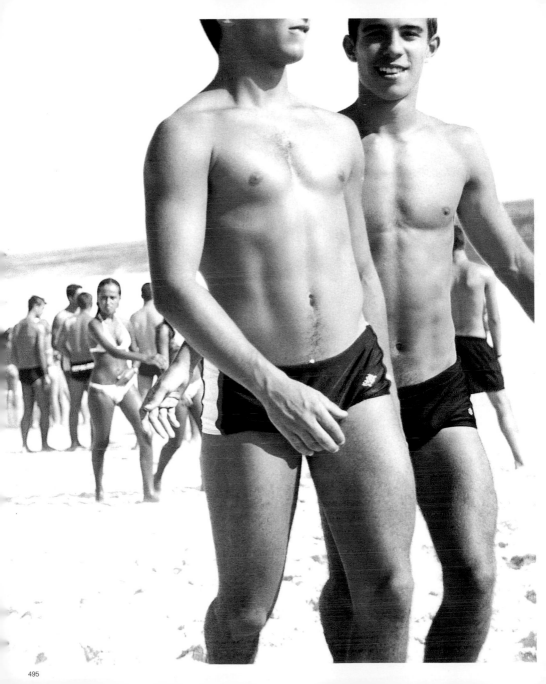

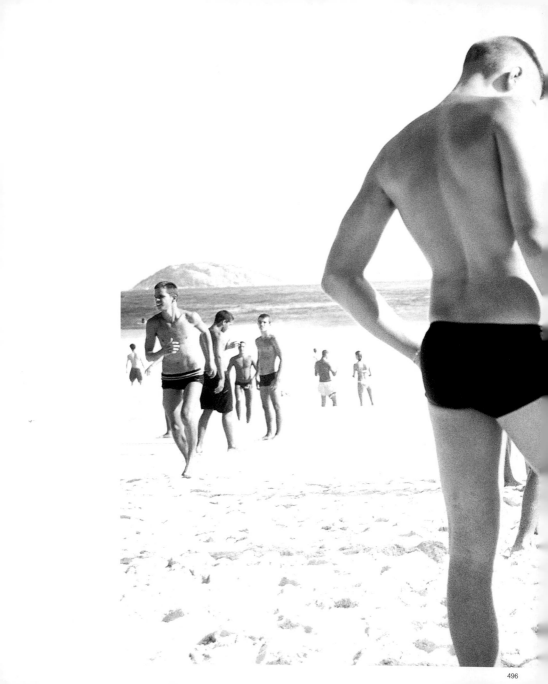

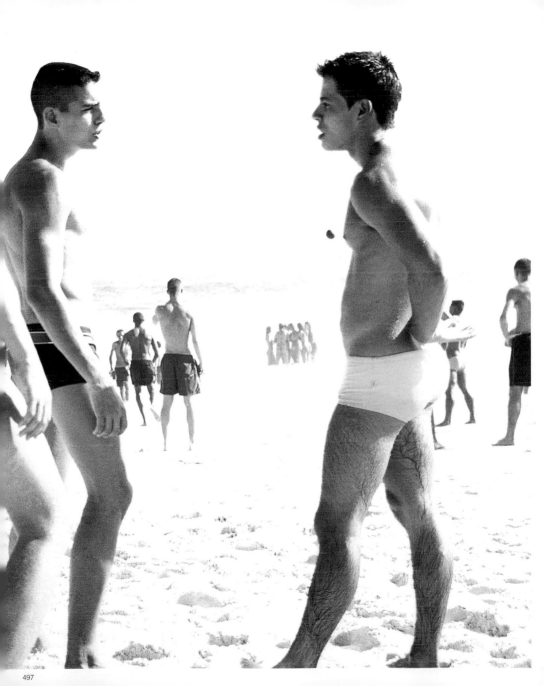

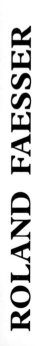

ROLAND FAESSER

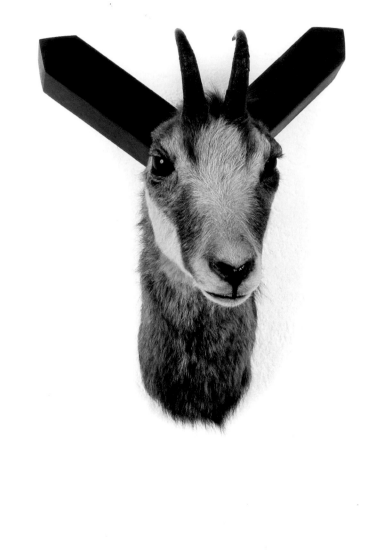

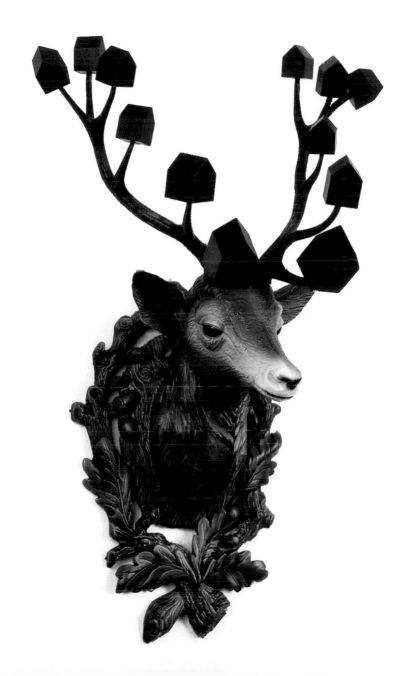

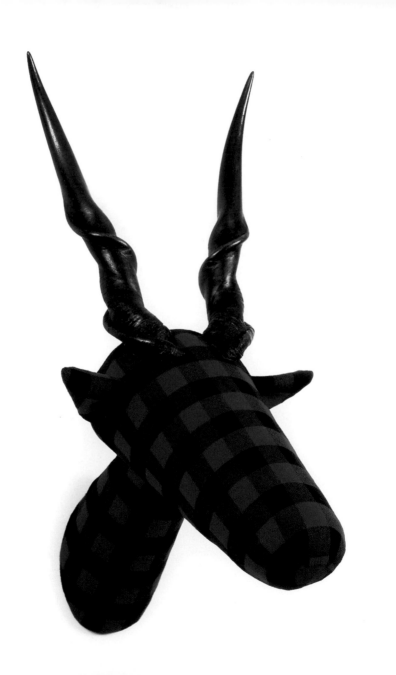

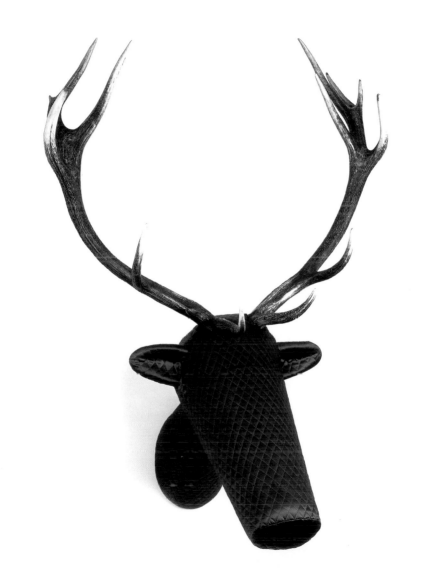

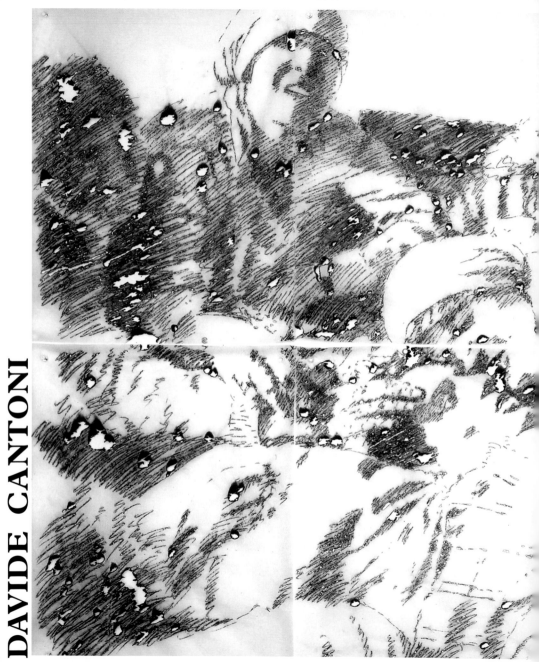

DAVIDE CANTONI

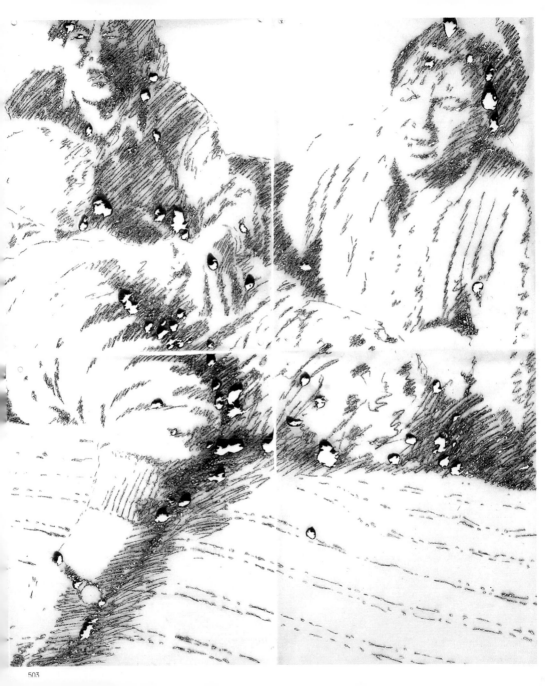

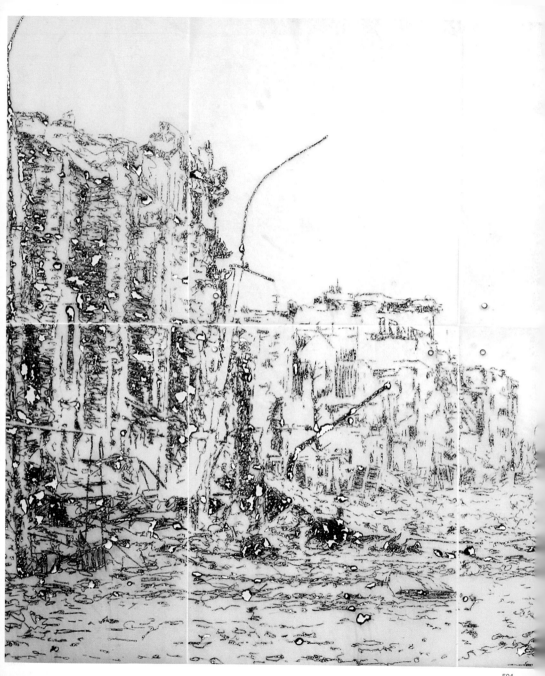

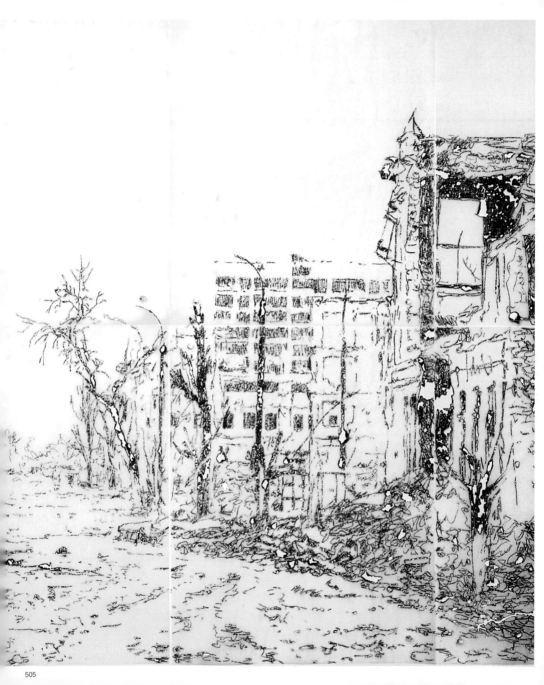

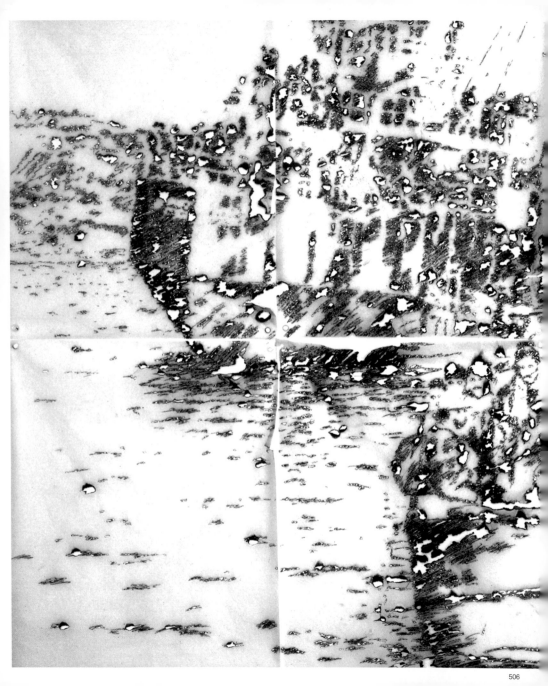

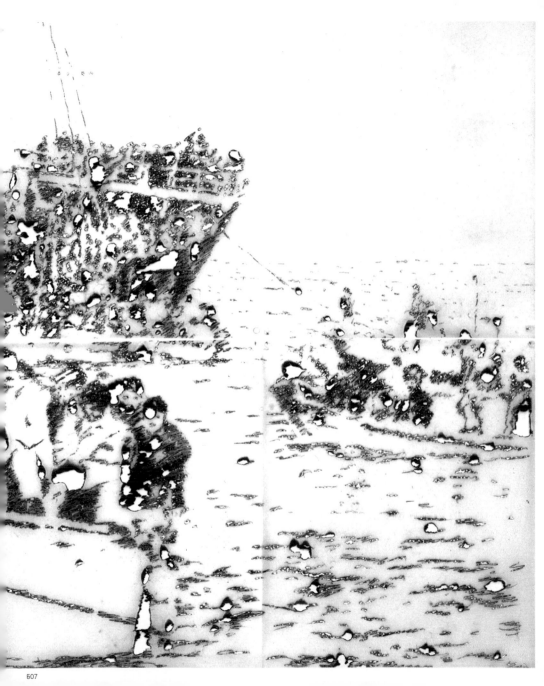

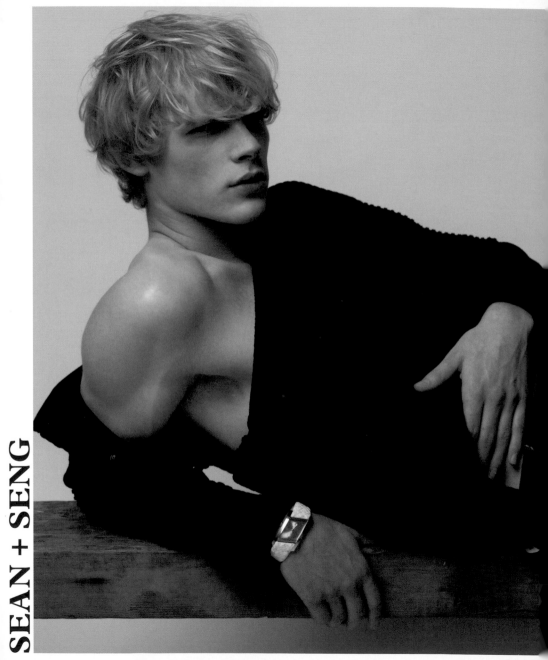

SEAN + SENG

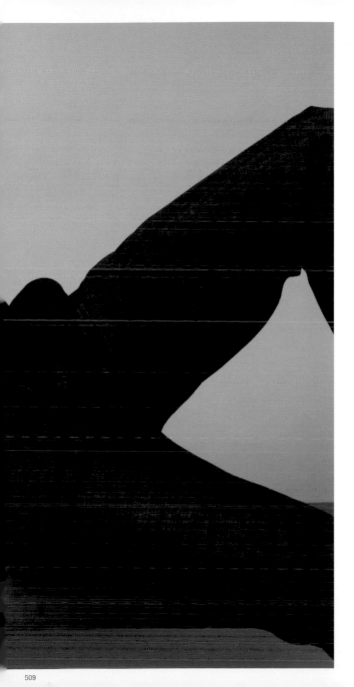

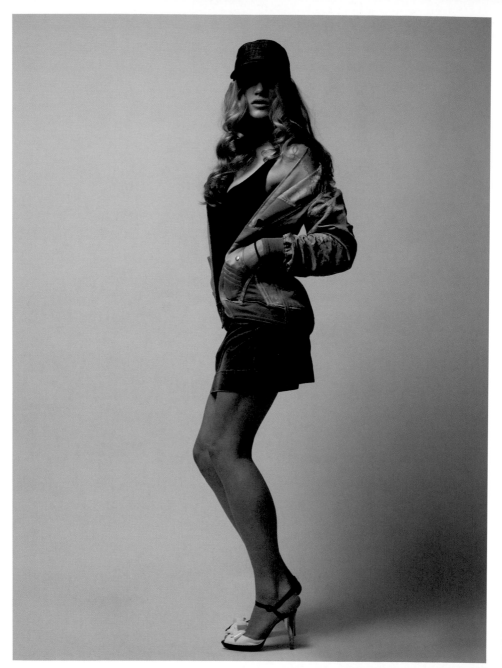

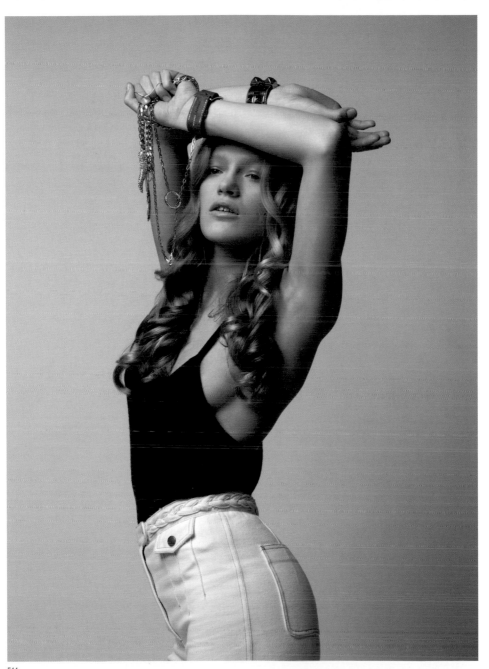

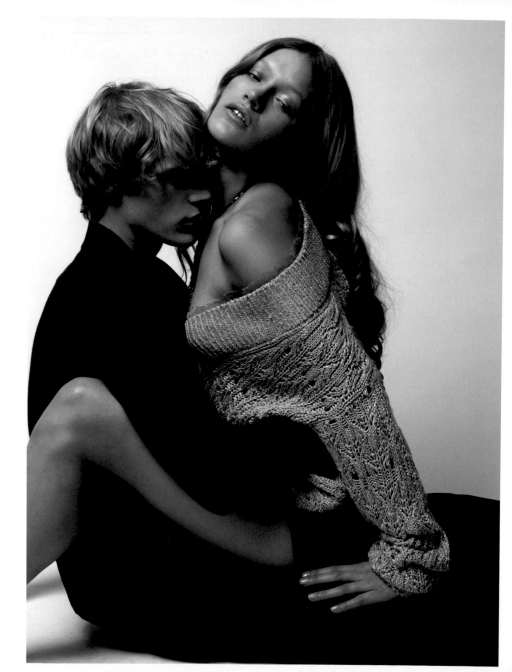

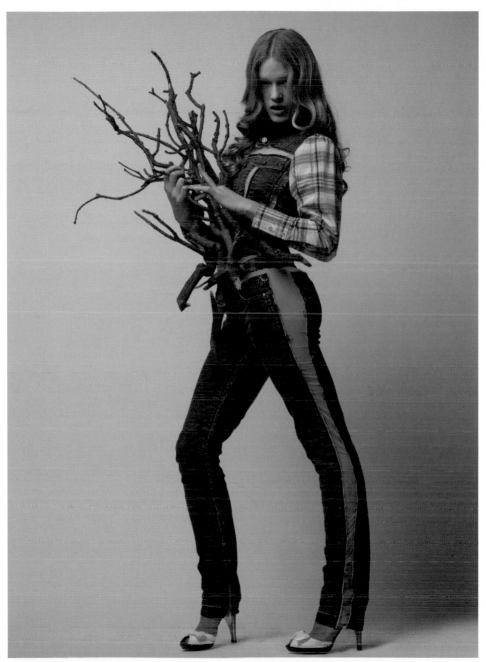

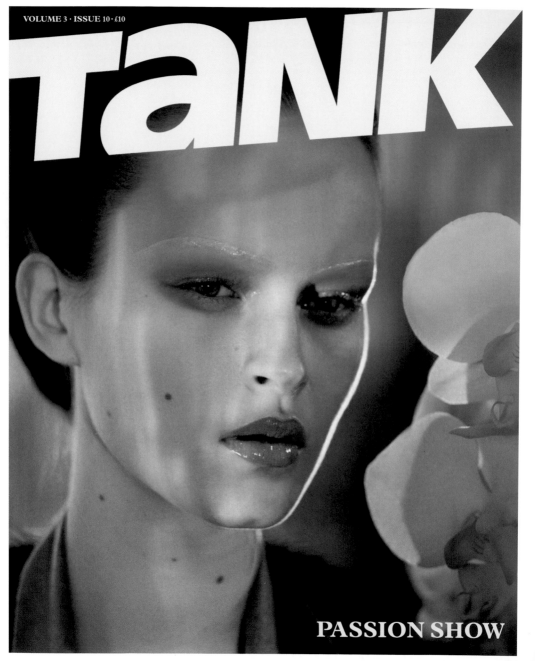

VOLUME 3 · ISSUE 10 · £10

TANK

PASSION SHOW

ART FELT

VOLUME 3 · ISSUE 10 · MAY 2004 · COVER PHOTOGRAPH BY STEFANO GALUZZI

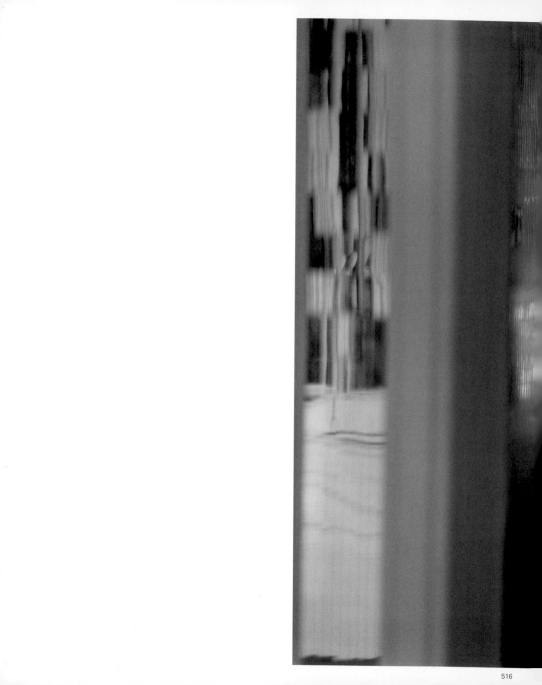

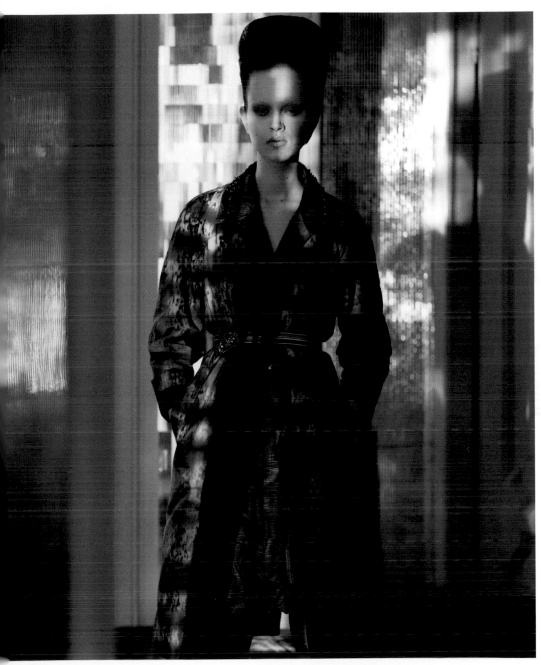

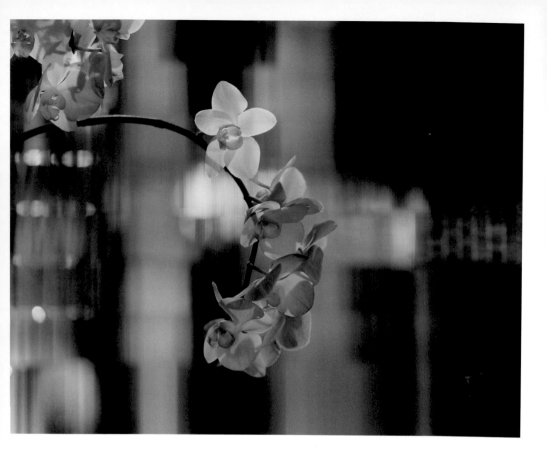

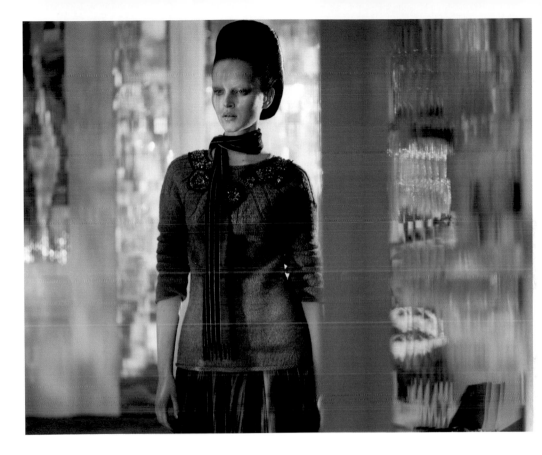

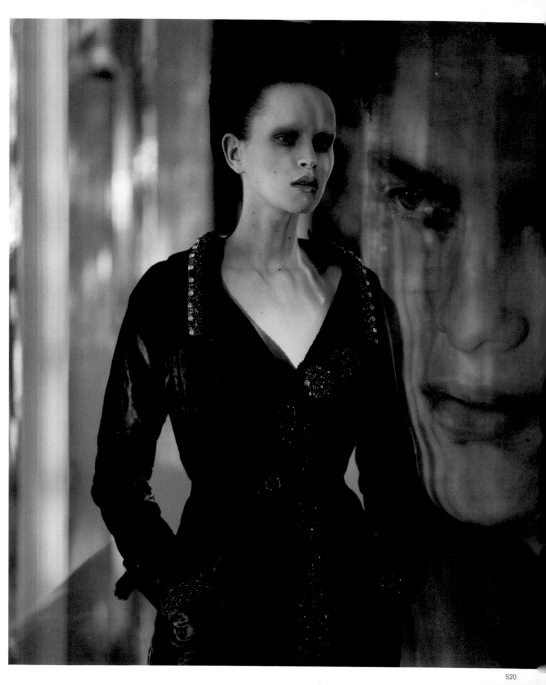

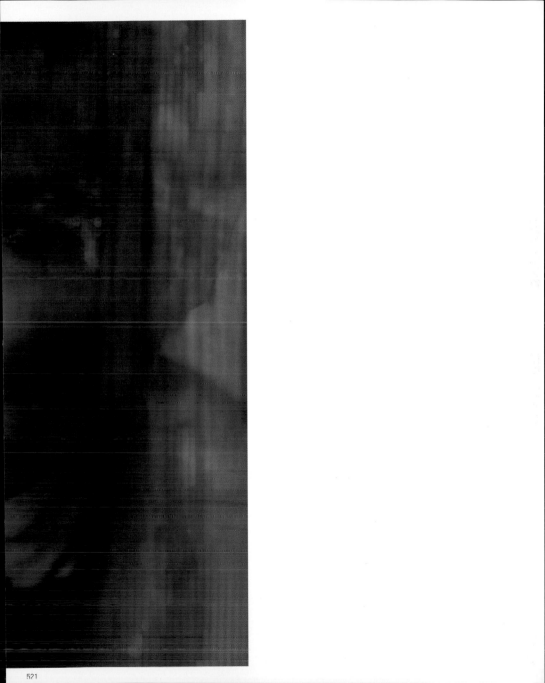

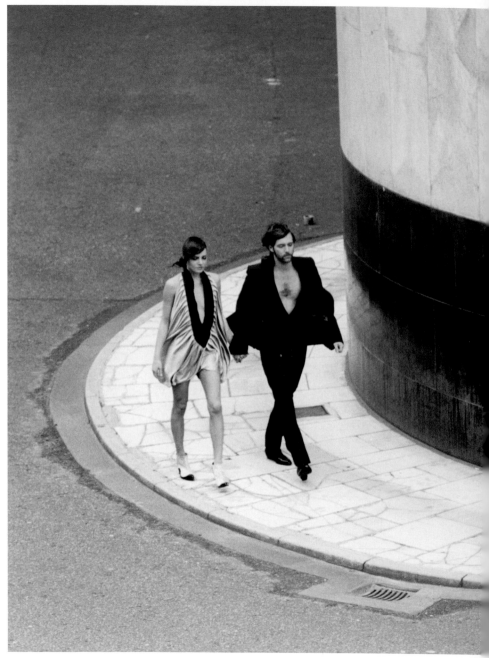

VALERIE STAHL

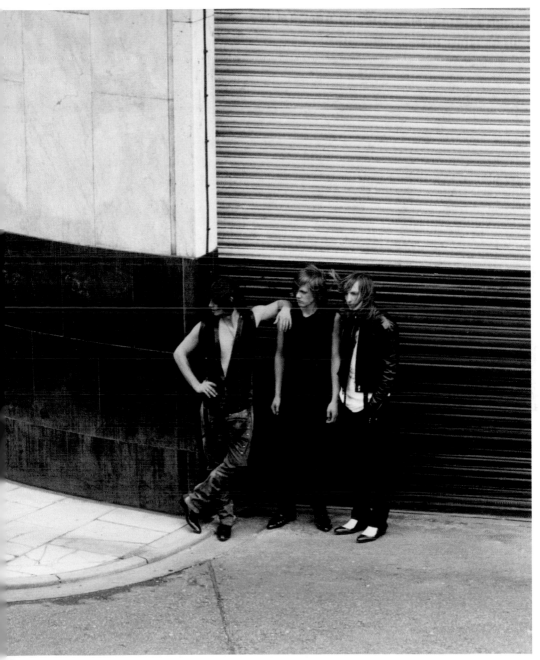

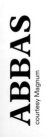

ABBAS
courtesy Magnum

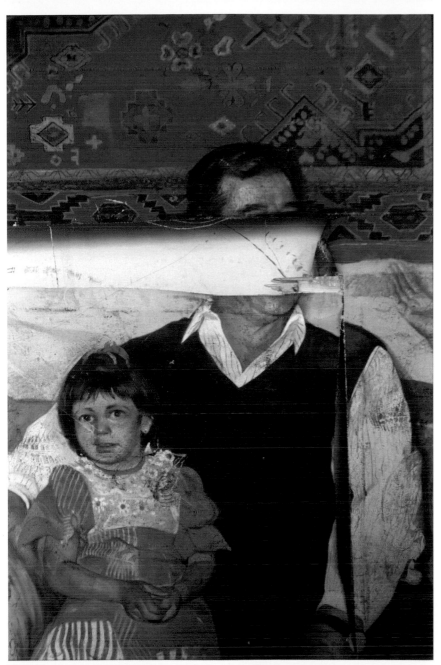

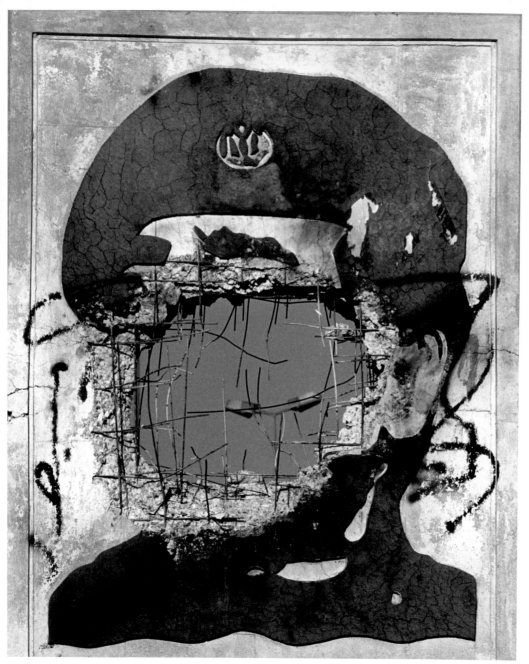

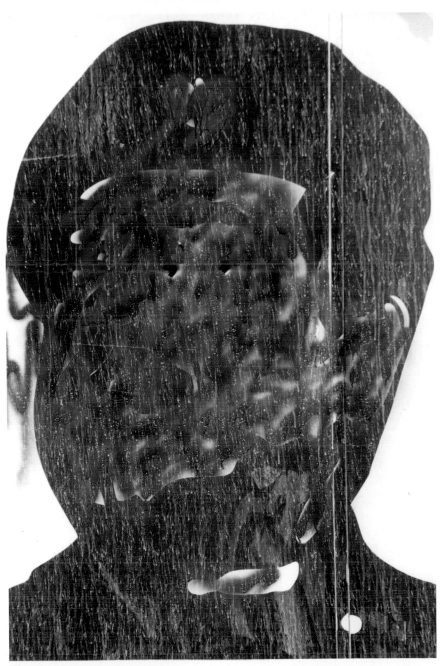

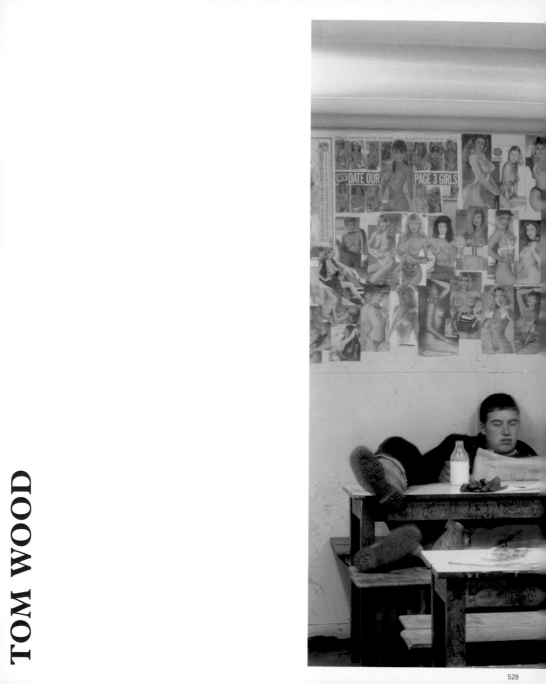

TOM WOOD

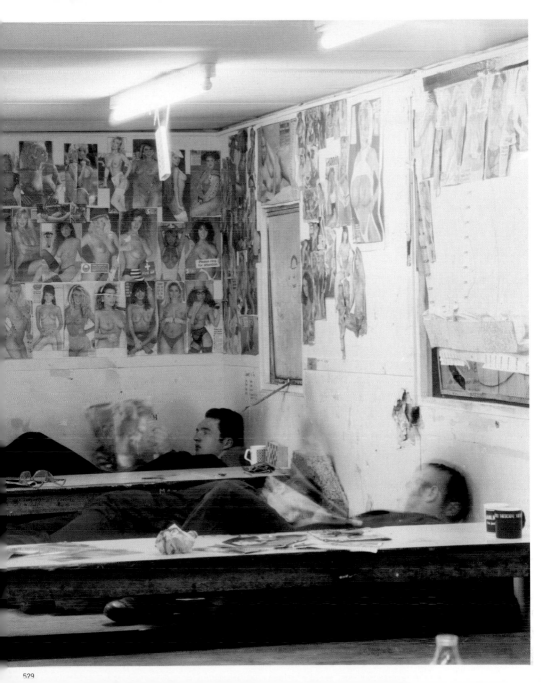

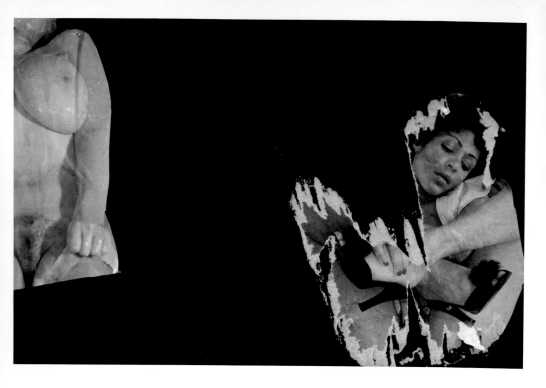

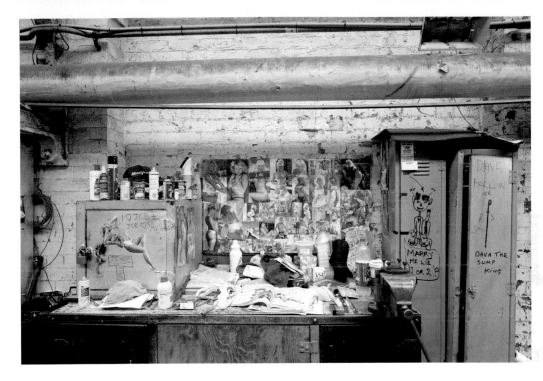

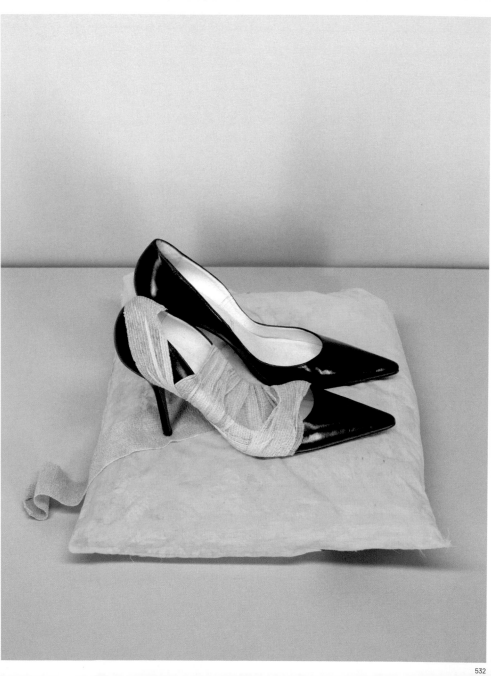

KATE PLUMB

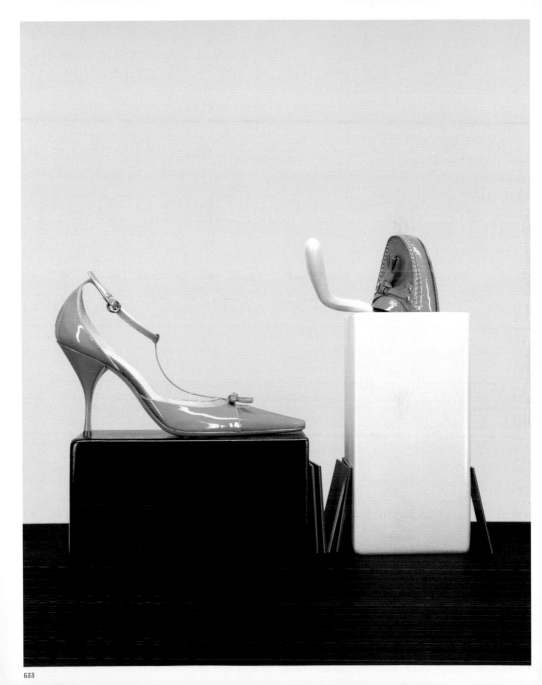

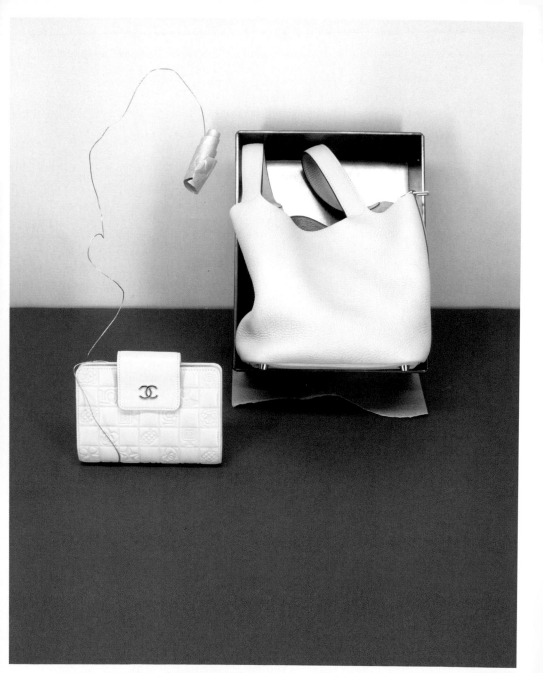

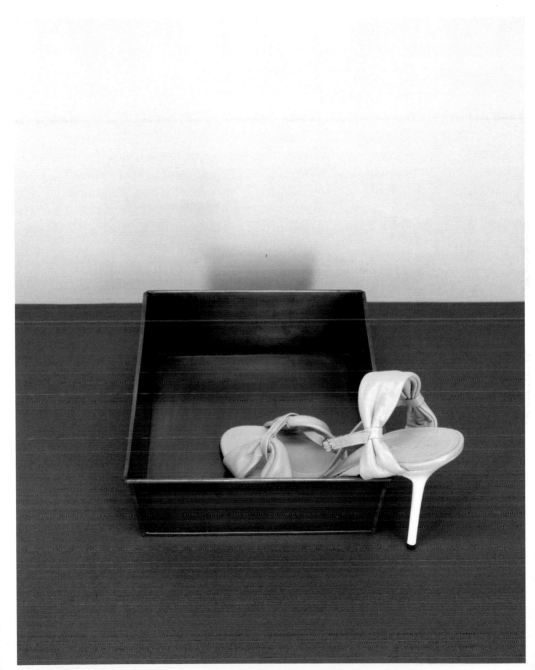

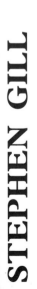

STEPHEN GILL

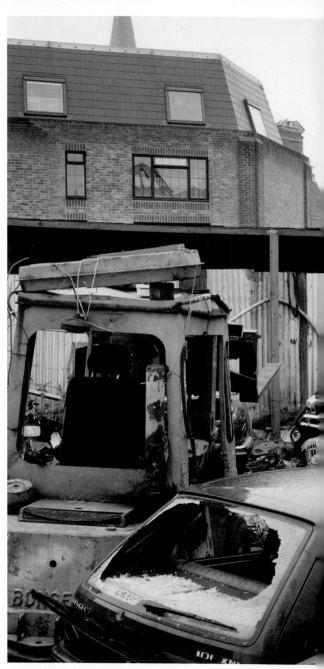

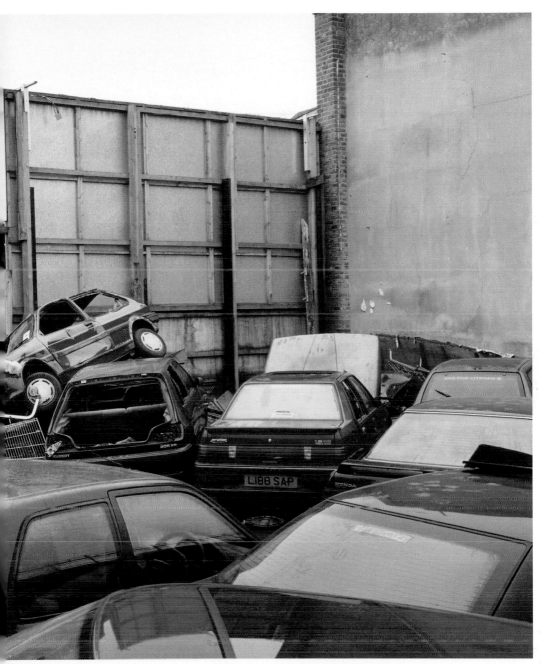

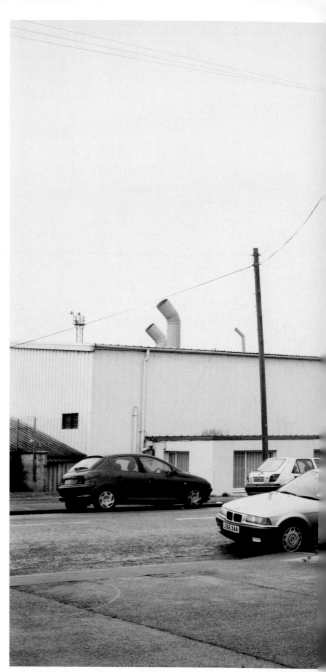

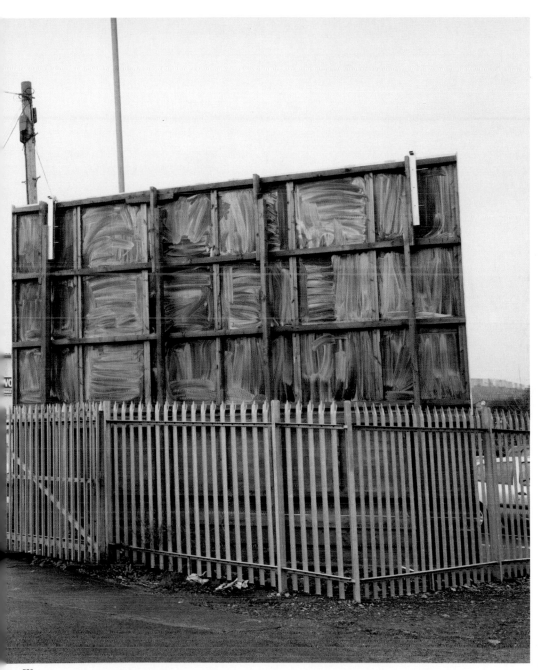

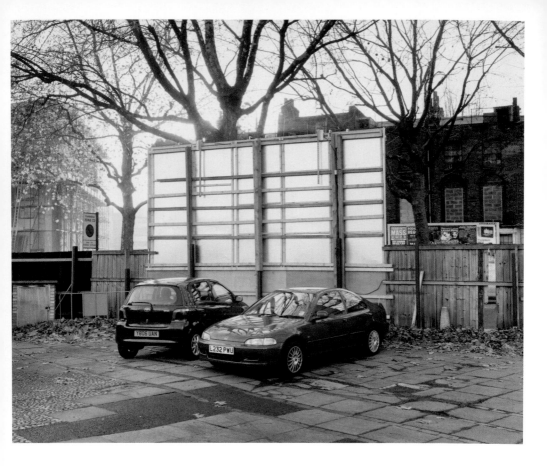

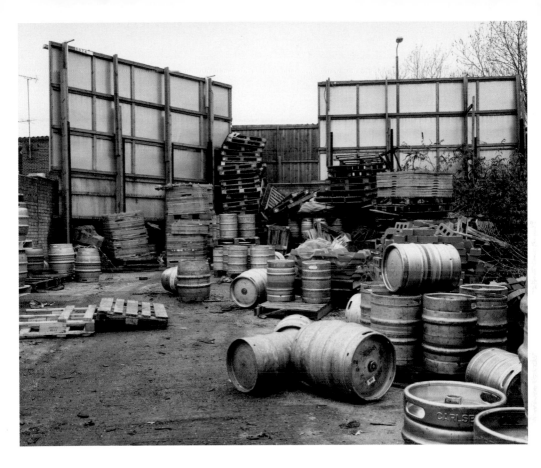

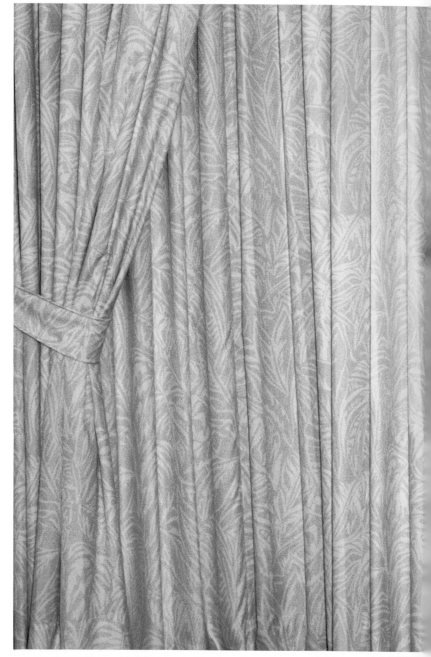

ANTONIO SPINOZA

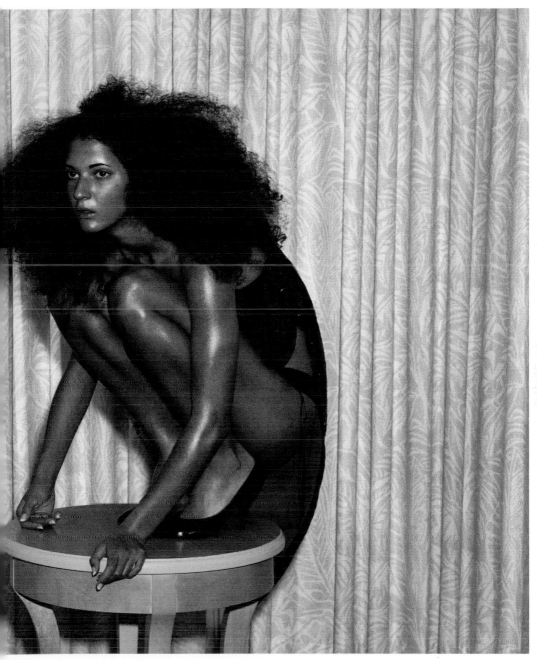

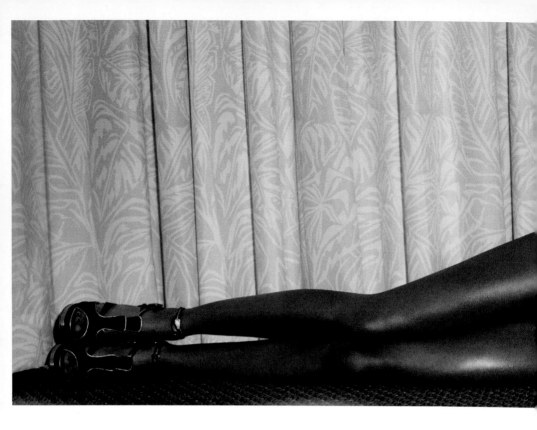

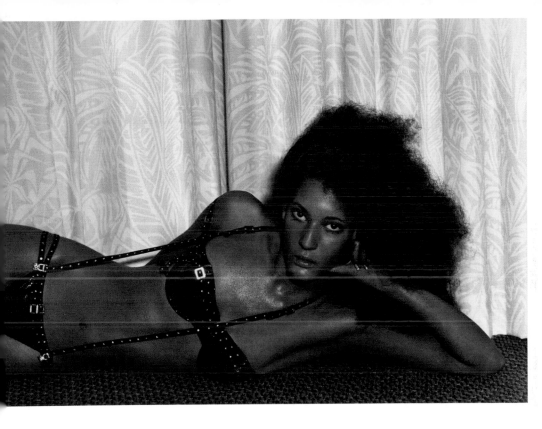

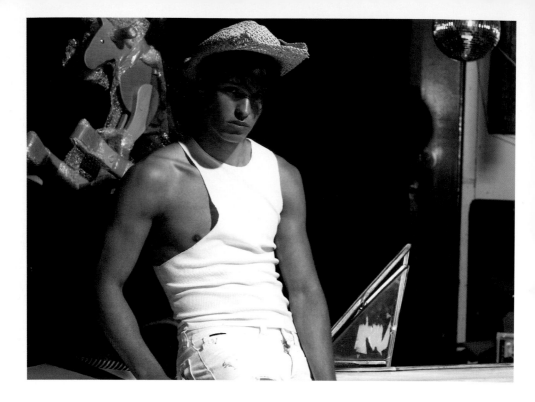

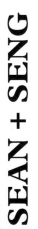
SEAN + SENG

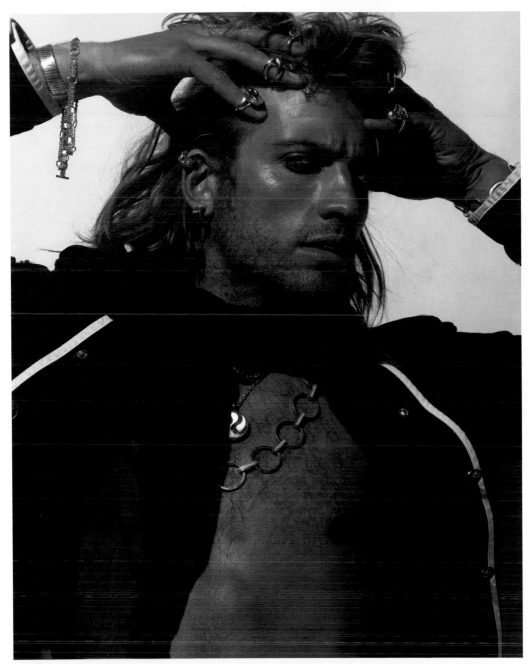

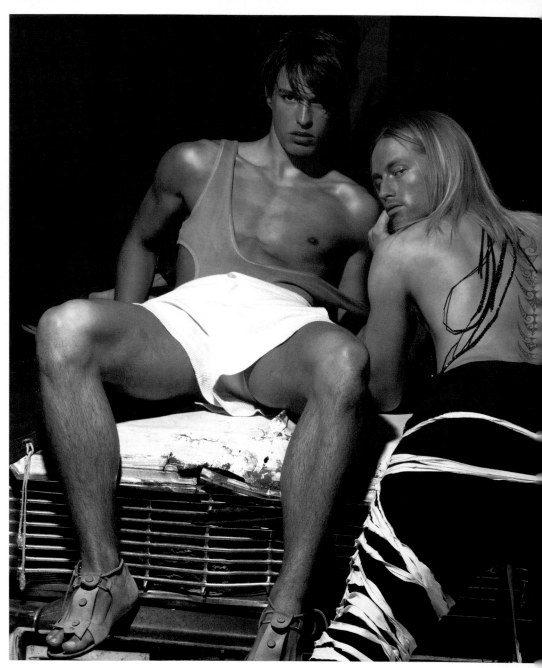

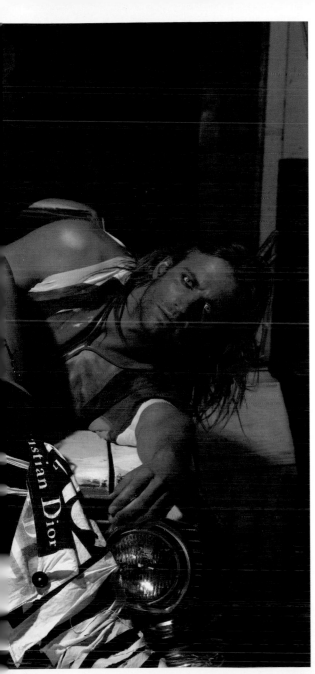

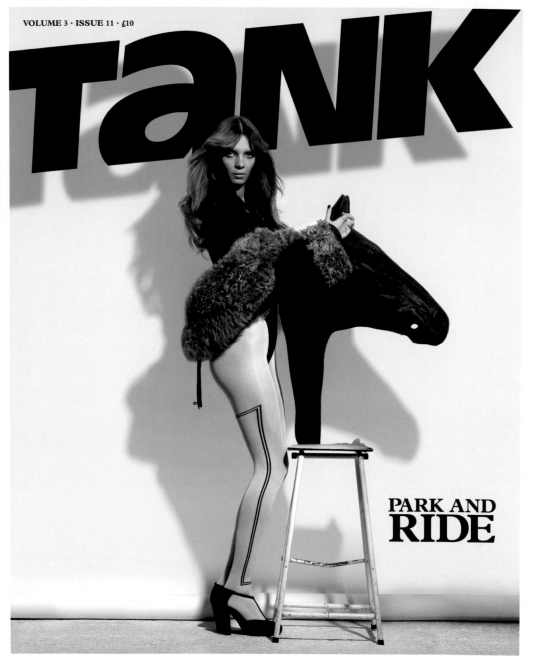

VOLUME 3 · ISSUE 11 · £10

TANK

PARK AND RIDE

PHOTO FINISH

VOLUME 3 · ISSUE 11 · SEPTEMBER 2004 · COVER PHOTOGRAPH BY SEAN + SENG

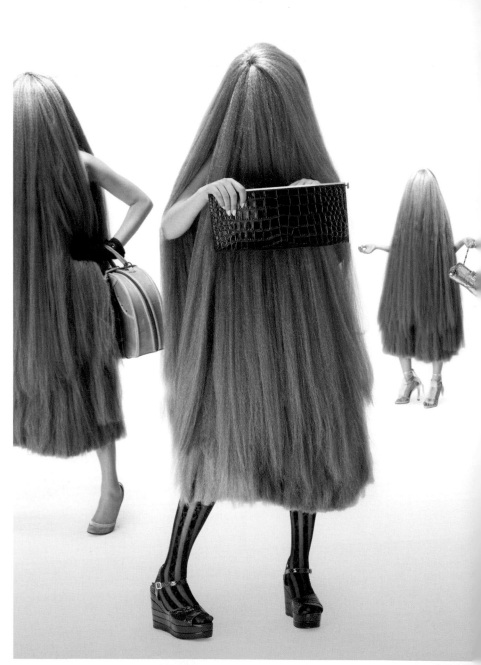

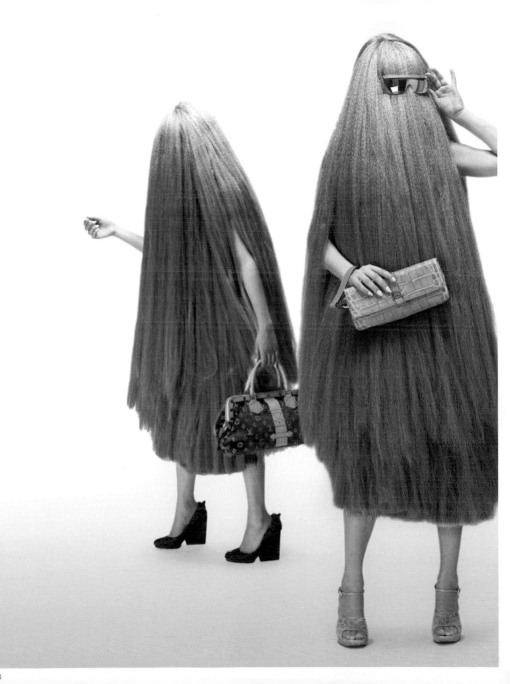

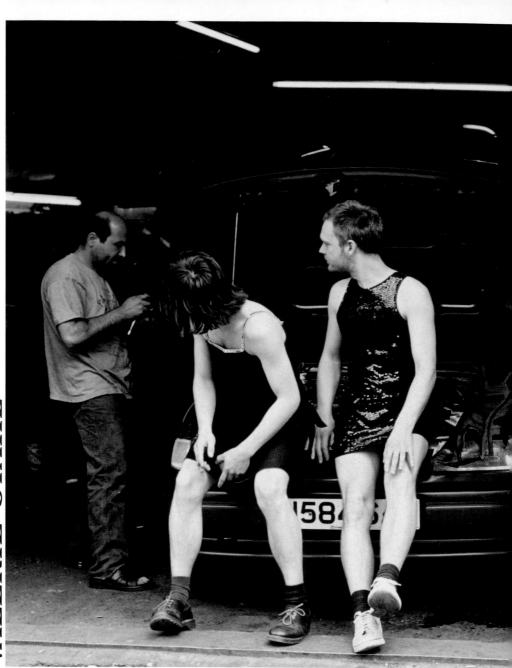

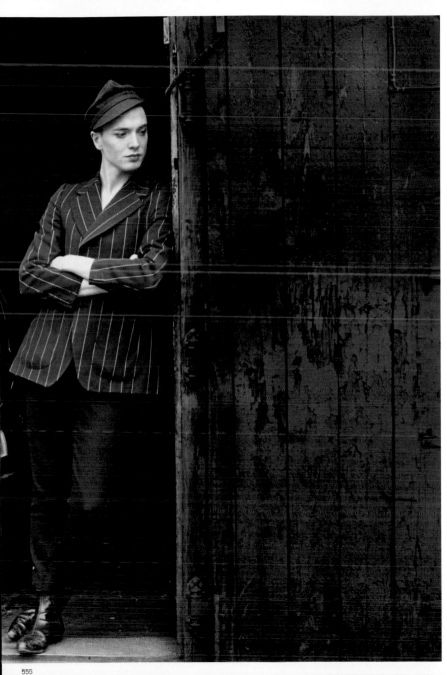

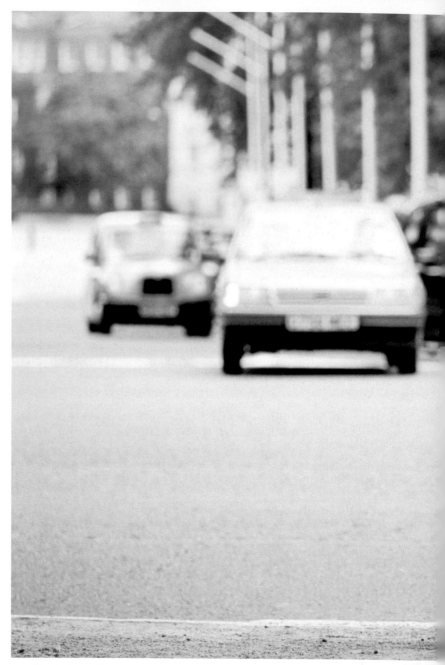

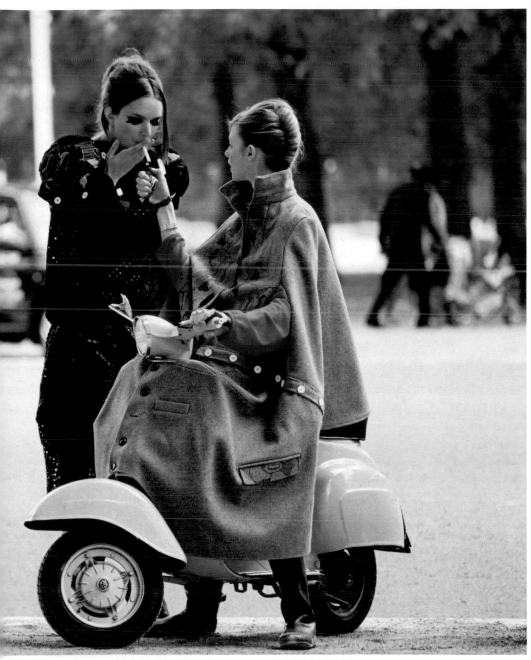

KATE PLUMB

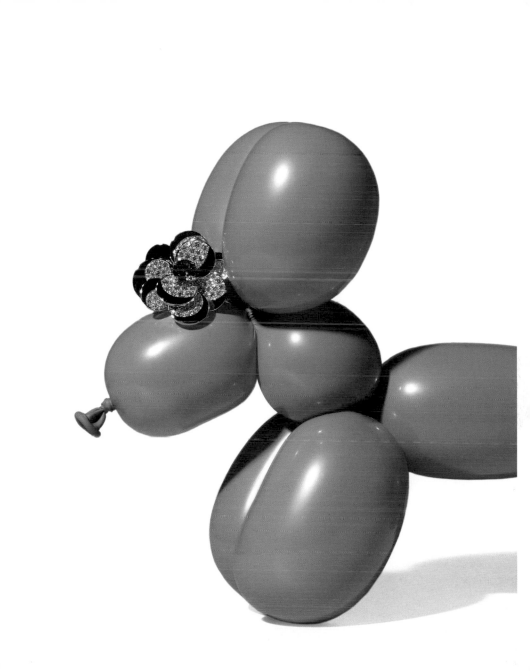

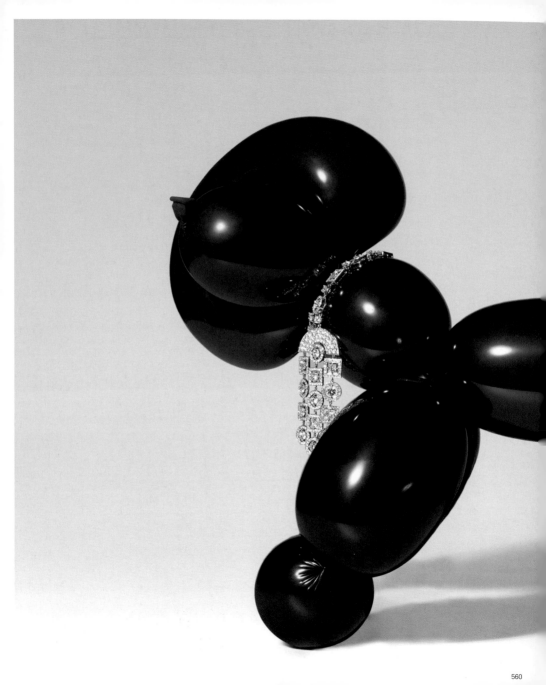

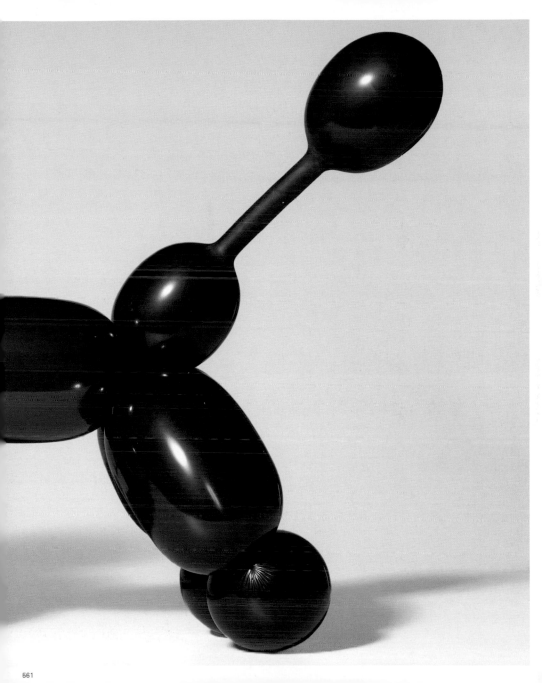

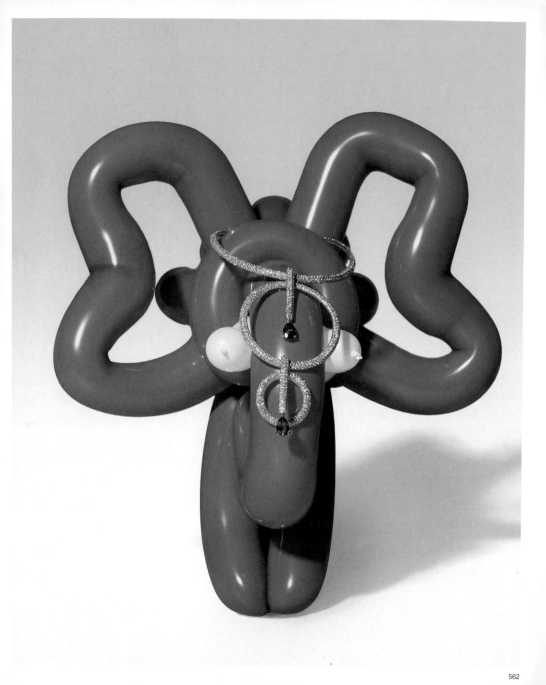

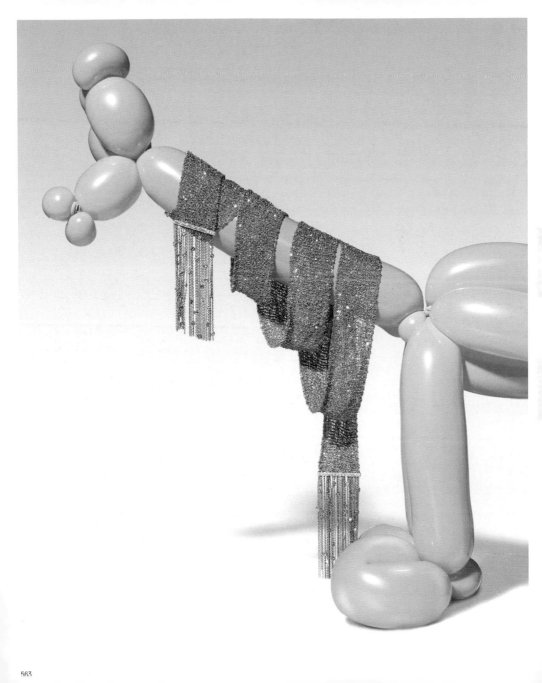

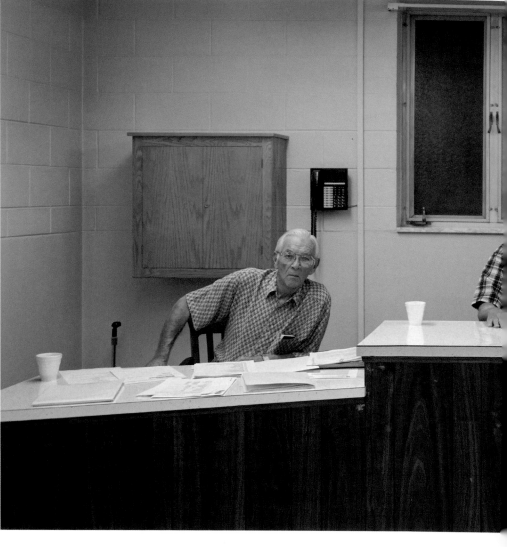

PAUL SHAMBROOM

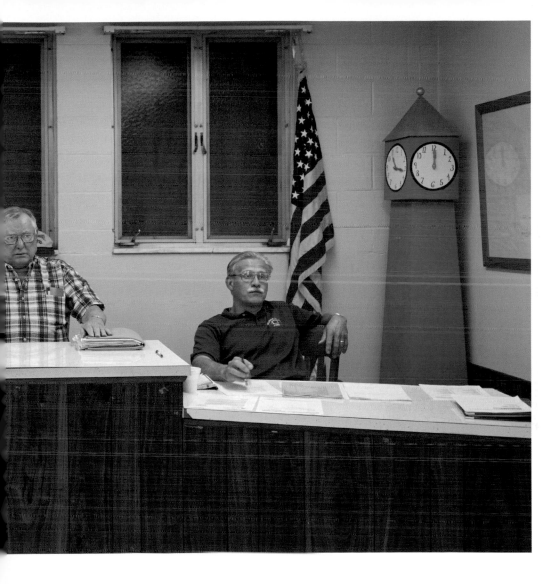

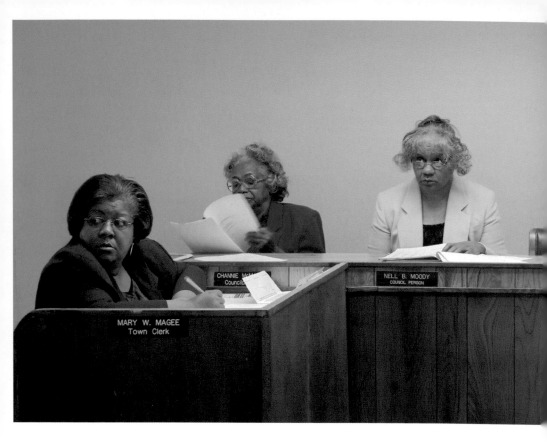

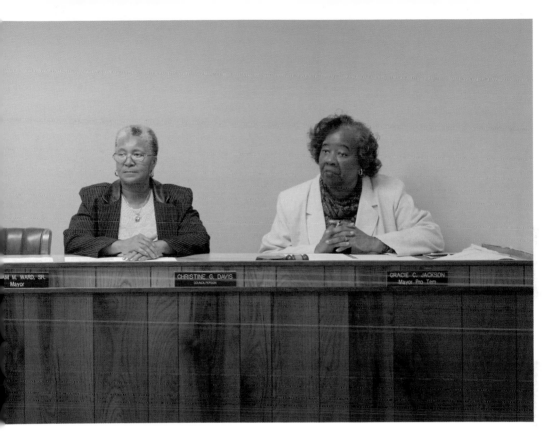

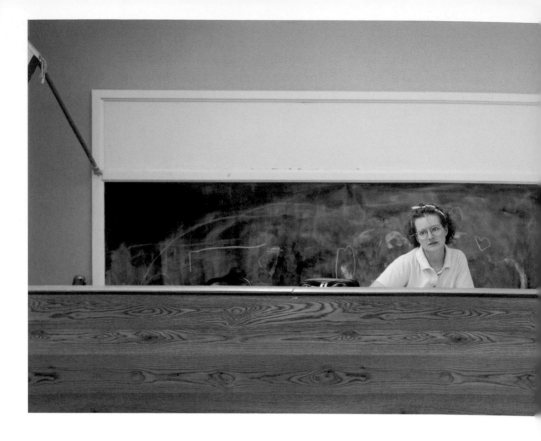

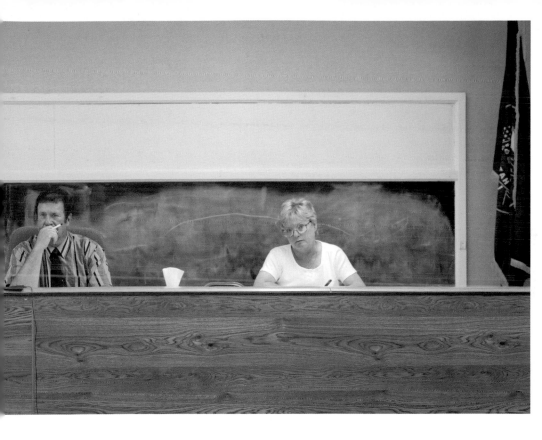

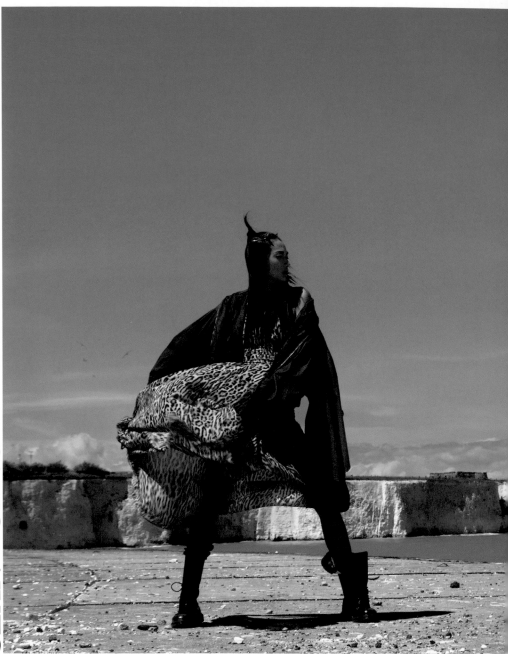

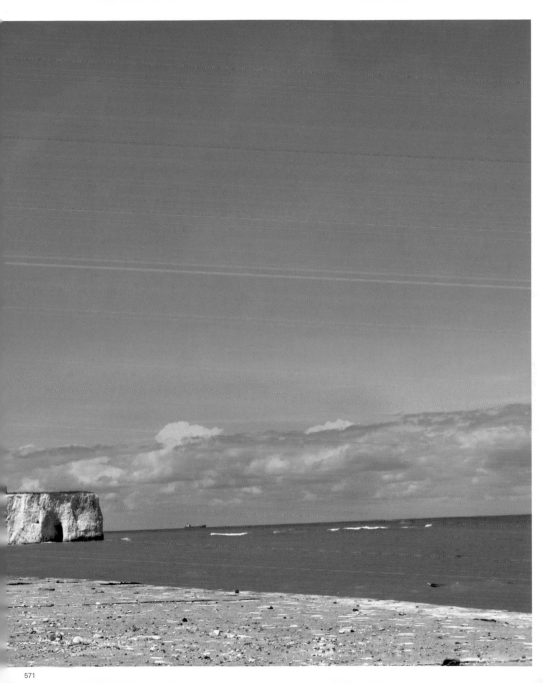

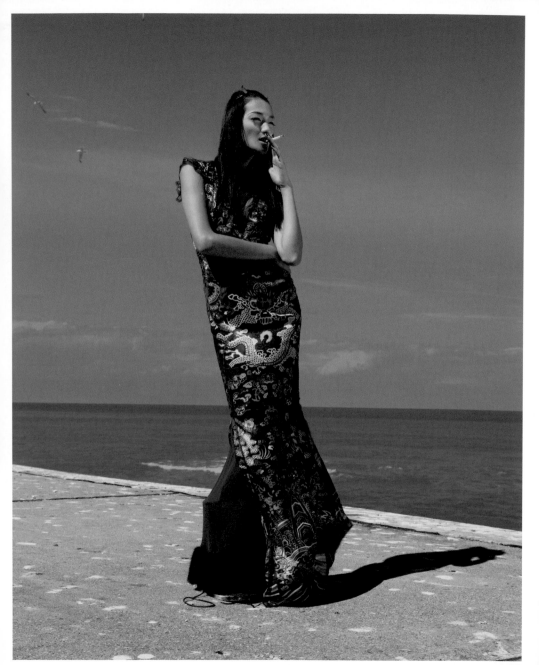

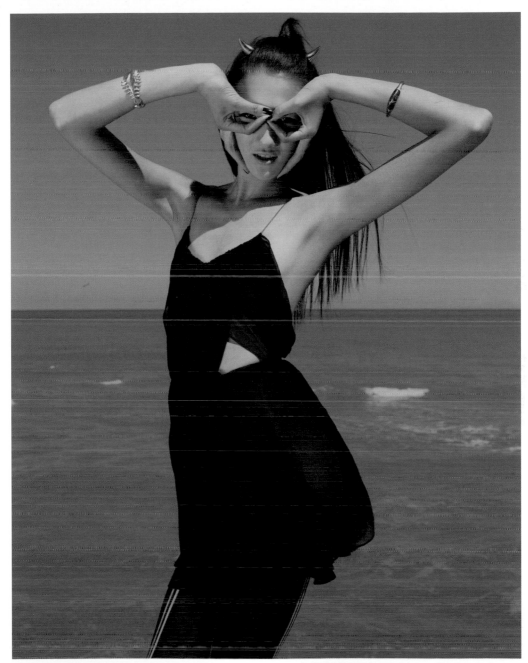

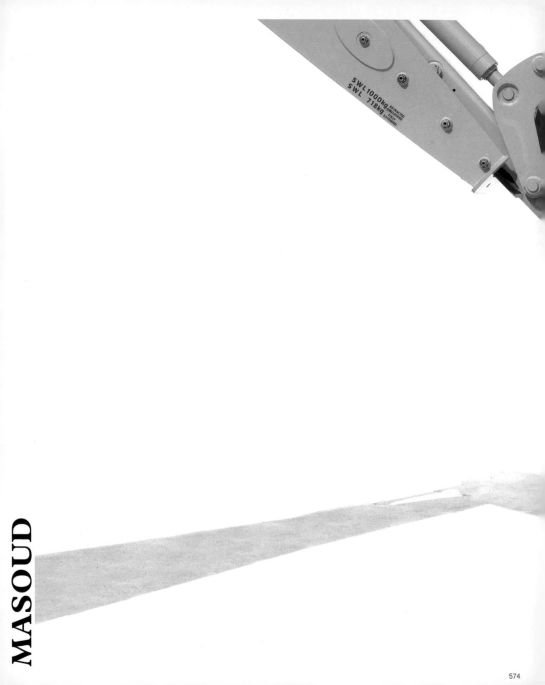

MASOUD

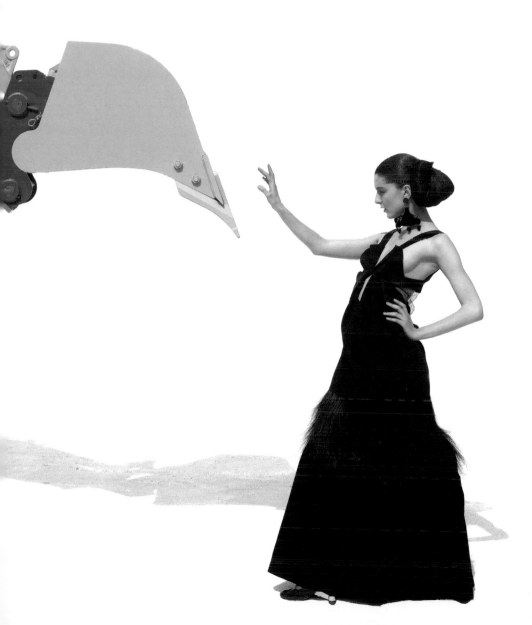

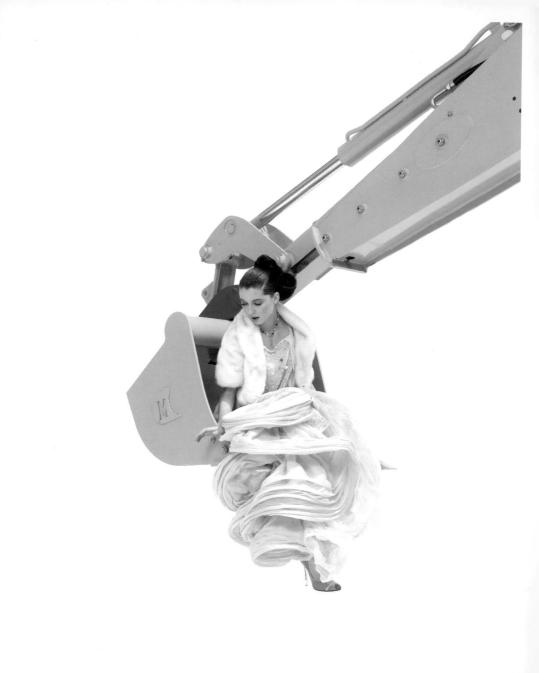

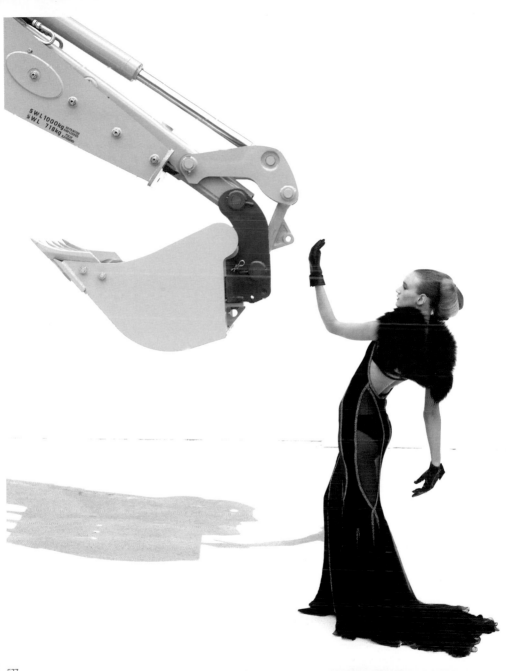

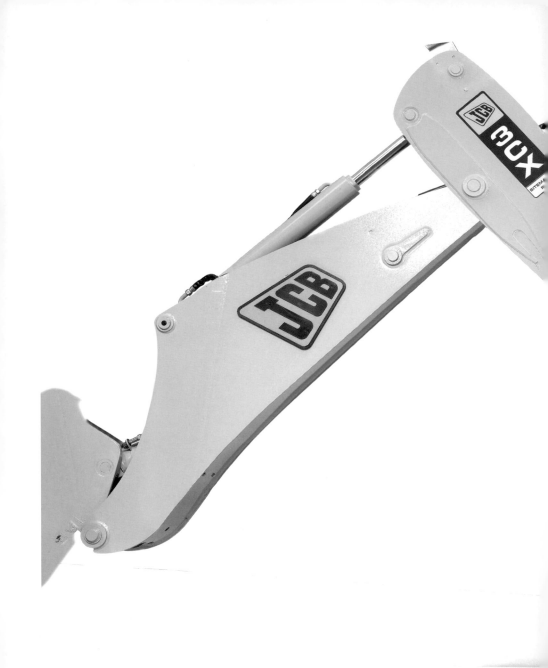

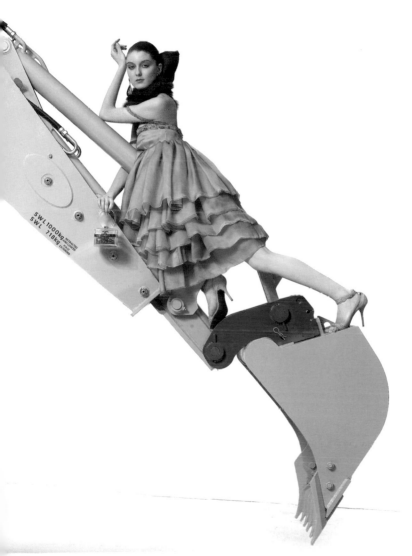

ELITISM FOR ALL
VOLUME 3 · ISSUE 12 · £10

TANK

People's **Democratic**
Republic of
Chic

REVELATIONARY

VOLUME 3 · ISSUE 12 · DECEMBER 2004 · COVER PHOTOGRAPH BY STEFANO GALUZZI

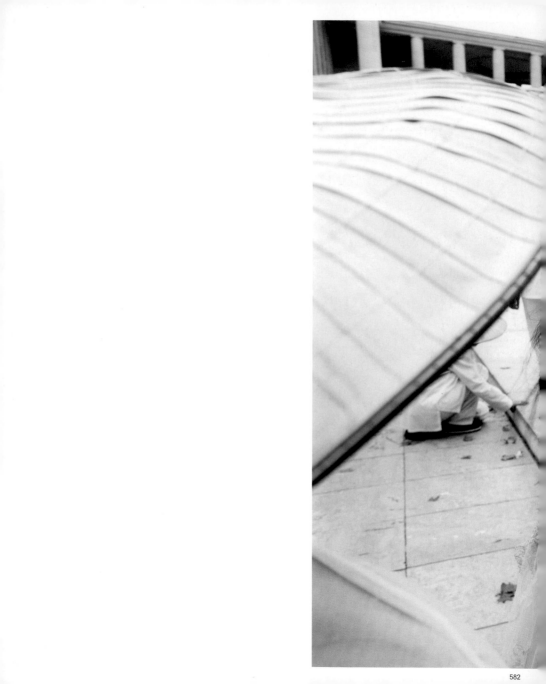

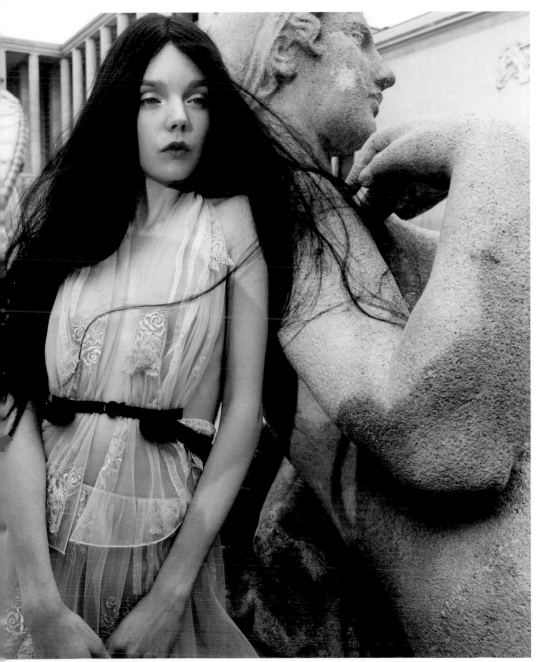

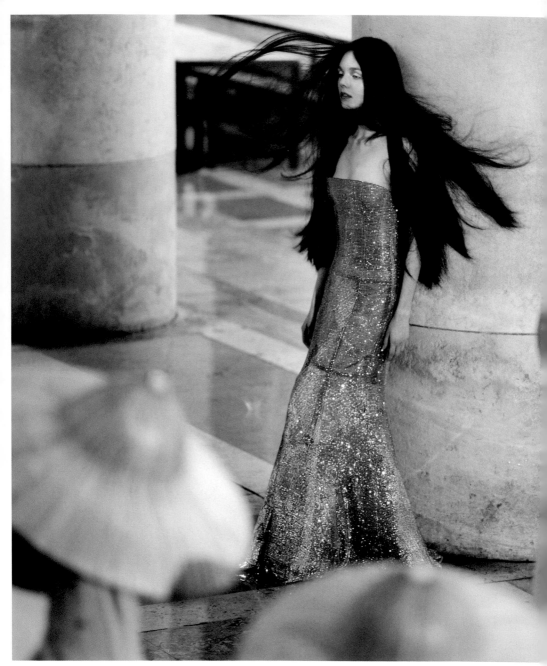

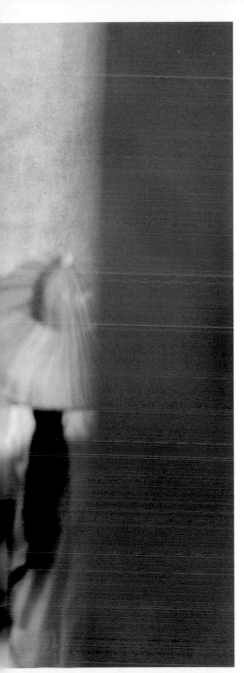

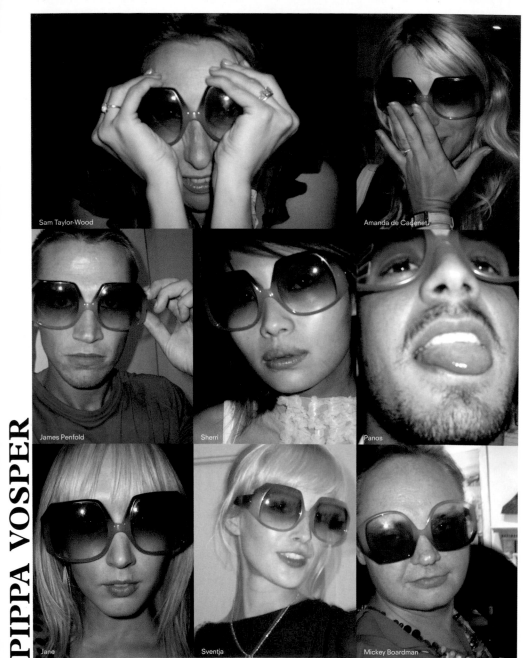

PIPPA VOSPER

Sam Taylor-Wood

Amanda de Cadenet

James Penfold

Sherri

Panos

Jane

Sventja

Mickey Boardman —

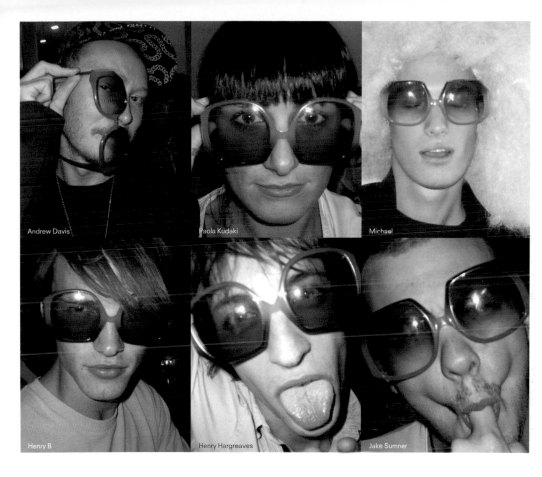

Andrew Davis

Paola Kudaki

Michael

Henry B

Henry Hargreaves

Jake Sumner

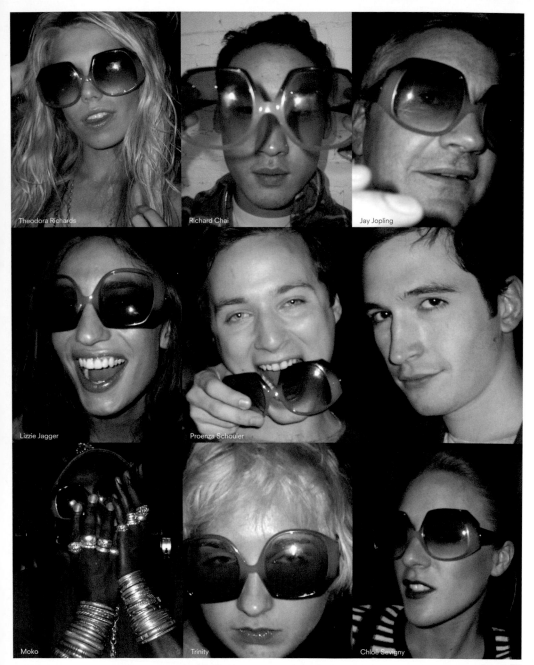

Theodora Richards

Richard Chai

Jay Jopling

Lizzie Jagger

Proenza Schouler

Moko

Trinity

Chloë Sevigny

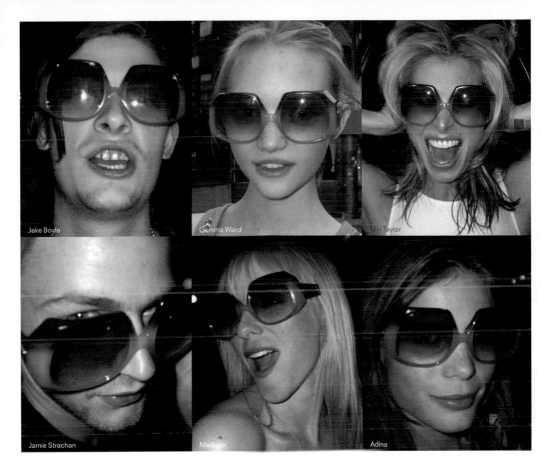

Jake Boyle

Gemma Ward

Niki Taylor

Jamie Strachan

Madison

Adina

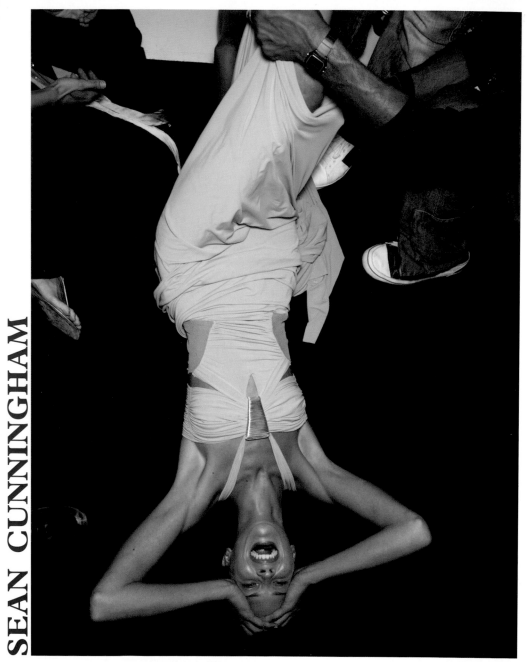

SEAN CUNNINGHAM

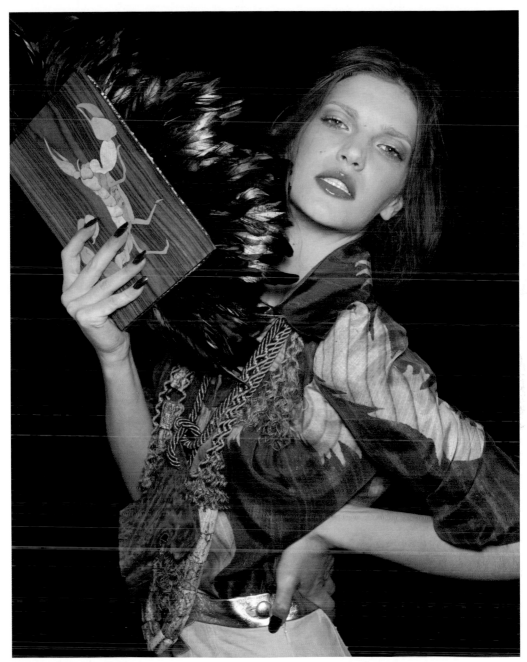

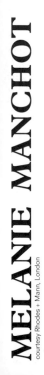

MELANIE MANCHOT

courtesy Rhodes + Mann, London

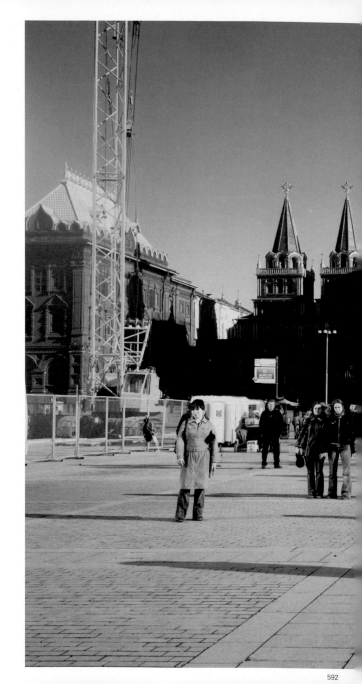

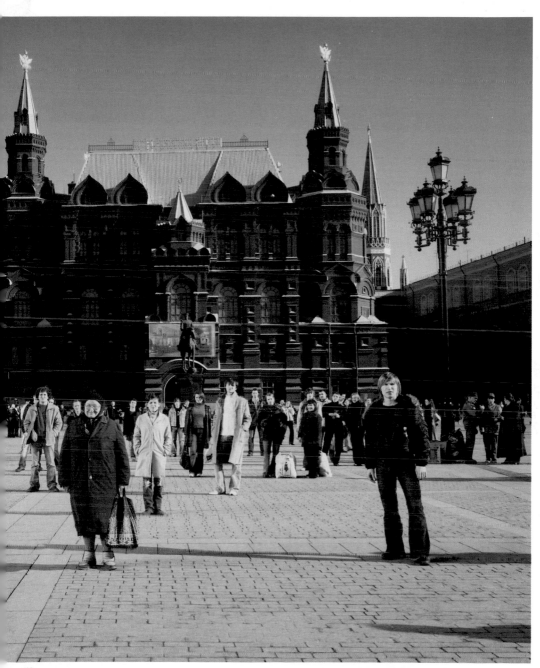

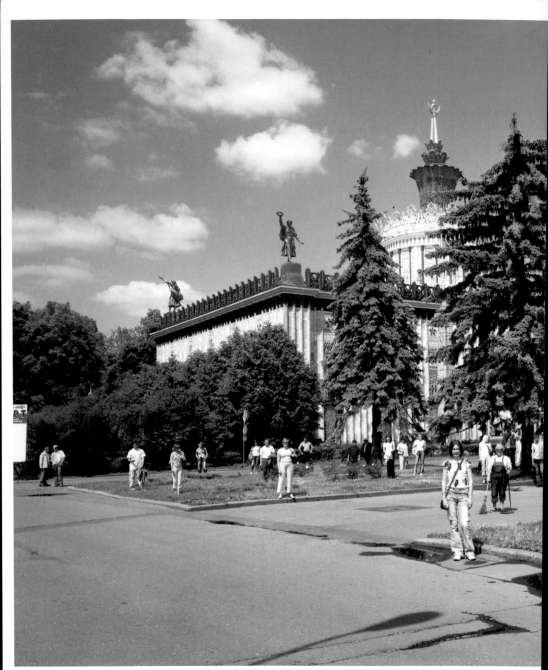

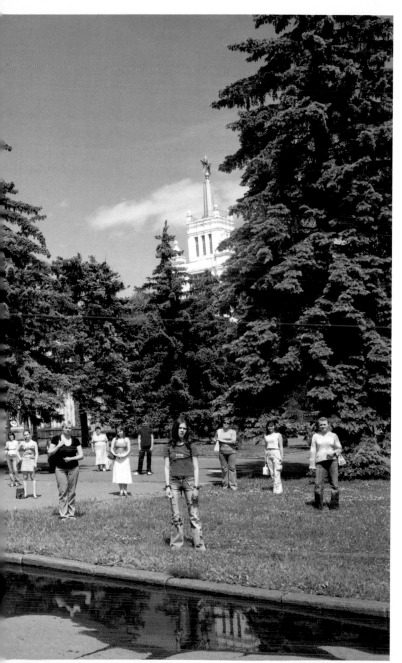

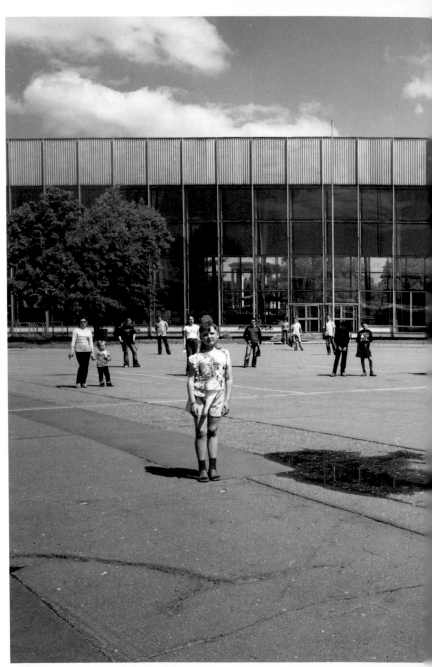

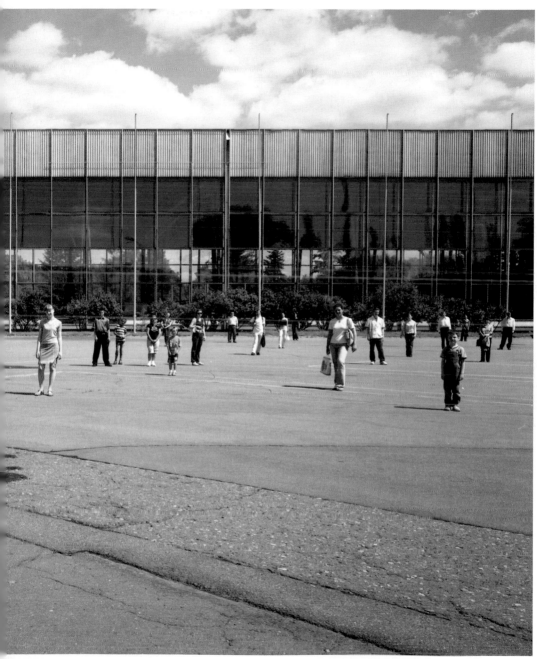

RAMMELLZEE

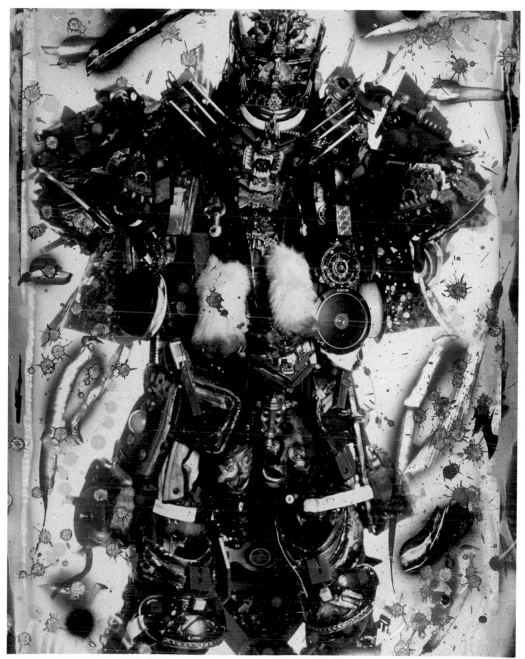

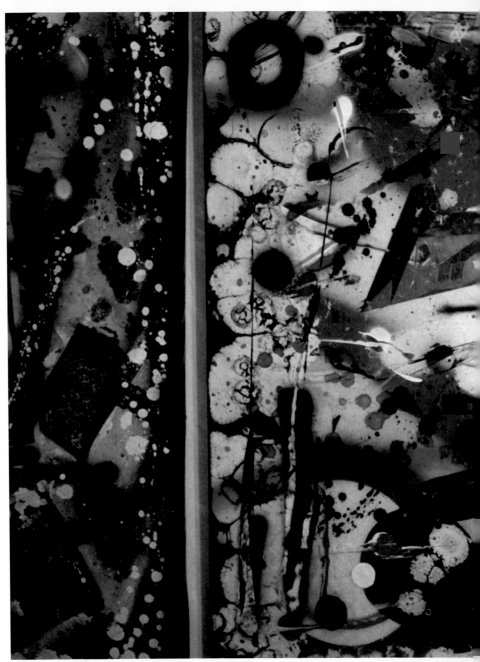

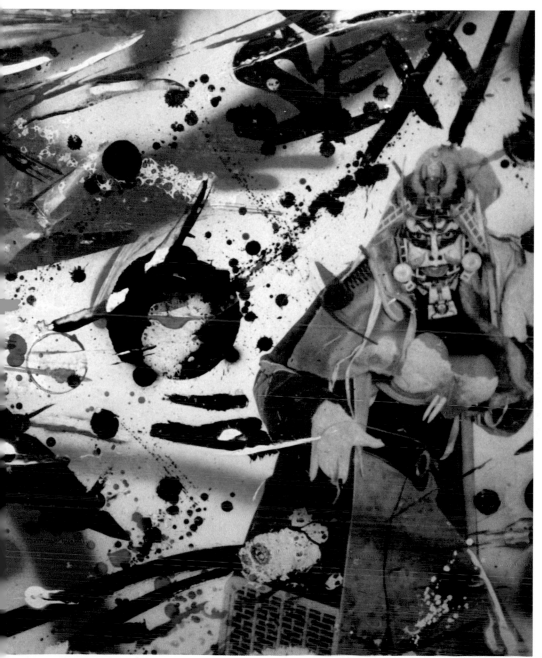

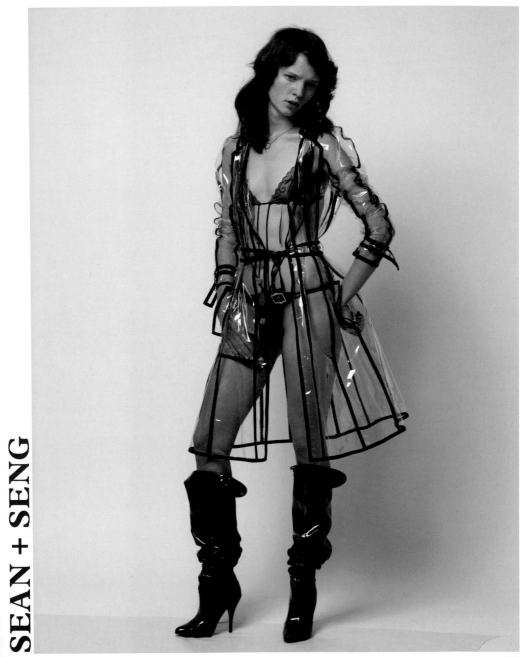

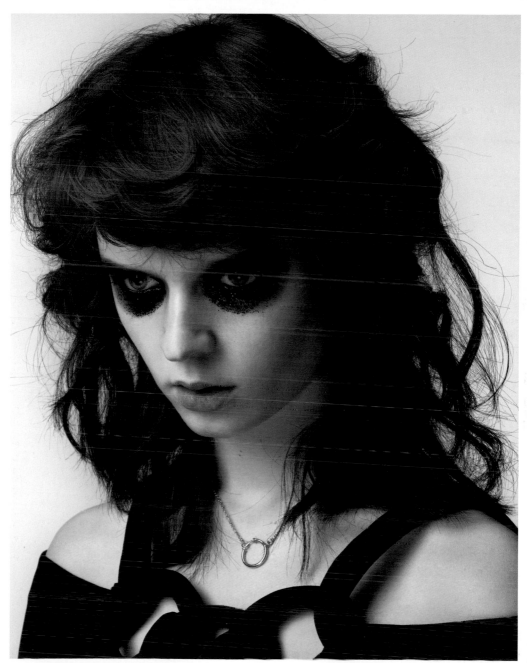

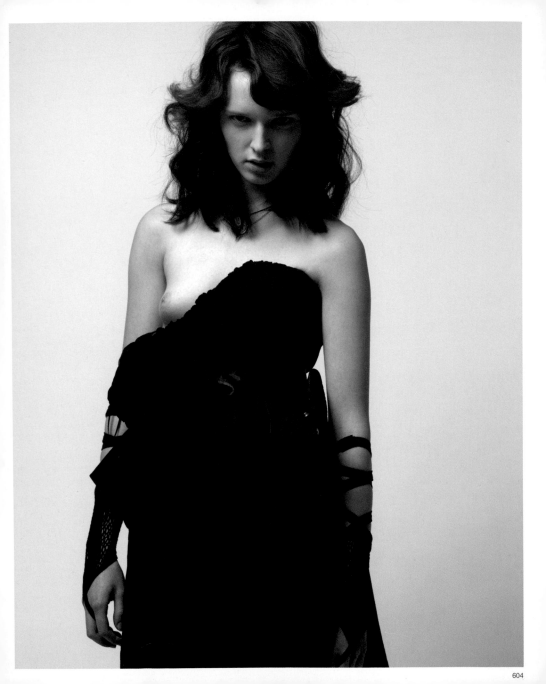

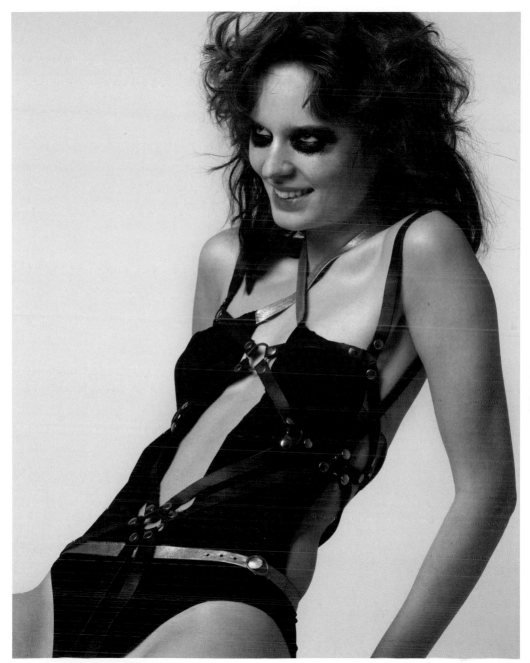

INDEX